The First-Time Parent's Guide to Potty Training

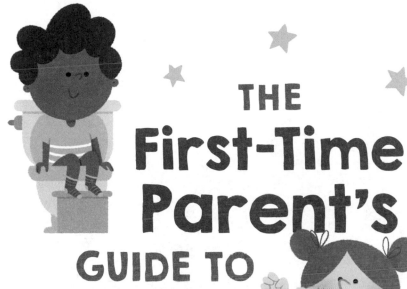

THE
First-Time
Parent's
GUIDE TO
POTTY
TRAINING

HOW TO
DITCH DIAPERS FAST
(AND FOR GOOD!)

Jazmine McCoy, PsyD
Illustrated by Marie Morey

ZEITGEIST • NEW YORK

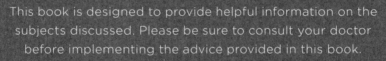

Published in the United States by Zeitgeist, an imprint of Zeitgeist™, a division of Penguin Random House LLC, New York.

penguinrandomhouse.com

Zeitgeist™ is a trademark of Penguin Random House LLC

ISBN: 9780593196663

Ebook ISBN: 9780593196731

Illustrations by Marie Morey

Book design by Aimee Fleck

Printed in the United States of America

3 5 7 9 10 8 6 4 2

First Edition

To my loving husband, Jessie, and our
two beautiful girls, Jayla and Jaliyah.

You all are the light of my life
and I love you so much.

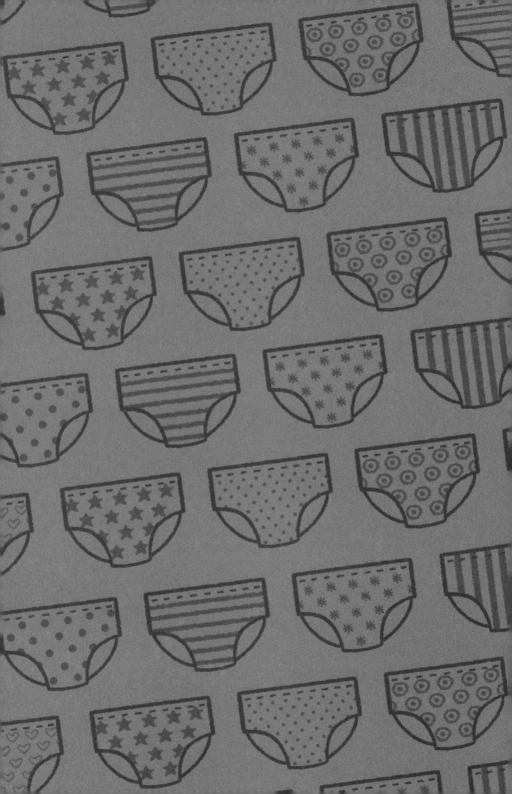

Contents

Introduction

POTTY TRAINING is a major milestone for both children *and* parents. It's the first time you get a clear look into *how* your child learns. It's also an opportunity for you to practice patience and trust in a process that is totally unfamiliar. As a clinical psychologist with an expertise in child development and positive parenting, and a mom of two children, I know how daunting potty training can be—especially for first-time parents who have never done this before! Luckily, it doesn't have to be this way. In fact, potty training can be an incredible opportunity to bond with your child and learn more about each other. Like any other milestone our children will face in life, this is one that can be embraced and celebrated.

It's normal to worry that you'll fail at potty training. You may wonder, *What if this doesn't work? What does that say about me as a parent?* And although diapers smell and are costly, they are much easier to deal with because *you're in control.* Potty training is a journey that requires you to place control in your child's hands. You teach them the skills, provide the structure, and empower and encourage them along the way, but then it's up to them.

I wrote this book with first-time parents in mind. I know how overwhelming and confusing it is to be faced with so much (often conflicting) information. This book puts all the pertinent information in one place to help you feel more prepared and confident to begin potty training. Plus, you'll find easy-to-read checklists throughout and a list of helpful books and DVDs at the end.

> **Potty training is a journey that requires you to place control in your child's hands.**

My program simplifies potty training and equips you with the tools and mindset you need to be successful throughout this process. You'll find important developmental milestones to consider when determining your child's readiness for potty training. You'll also learn how to prepare for the big event and how to set ground rules. In addition, there is important information about naps and nighttime training and how to navigate your child's personality traits, developmental delays, and other unique situations that may affect the process. Perhaps most importantly for today's busy parents, you'll learn about potty training while on the go and in day care and other caregiving situations, as well as how to troubleshoot common issues such as temper tantrums and regression.

Keep in mind that one size does not fit all in potty training. Every child is unique, and developmental milestones play a huge role in the success (or setbacks) of potty training. Furthermore, children have their own thoughts and opinions. They ultimately call the shots here, but *you* make all the difference in how this process goes. You are their teacher. You provide safety and boundaries, as well as a loving environment in which they will thrive. I'm here to empower you in your role and help you navigate this uncharted territory. You *will* succeed, and your child *will* be potty trained. I will be here every step of the way, with practical and positive suggestions to help make the process more intuitive and fun.

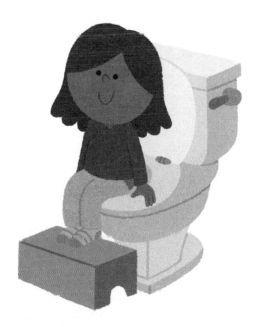

Before You Begin

As a first-time parent, you might not realize that potty training requires some forethought. Is your child ready to start? Have they reached the necessary developmental milestones? Have you bought the necessary equipment (like a potty chair)? Do you have a thorough understanding of what lies ahead for both you and your child? Here's what you need to know to be prepared for the big event.

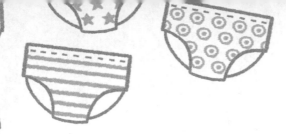

CHAPTER 1

Is Your Child Ready? Are You Ready?

UNFORTUNATELY, THERE'S NO MAGICAL AGE for potty training. However, children send subtle signals that they're ready as they reach certain developmental milestones. Once you know the physiological, motor, cognitive, verbal, and emotional/social signs that your child is ready to learn to use the toilet, you'll be able to prepare mentally for this transition.

Ages and Stages

Children in the United States are generally potty trained between 21 and 36 months of age. Nearly one-third of children achieve daytime potty training by 24 months, and most achieve it by 36 months. On average, girls tend to master potty training 2 to 3 months earlier than boys. Remember, though, it's more important to focus on your child's developmental progress than on their age. After all, each child is different and will achieve potty training in their own time.

There are benefits and drawbacks to both potty training early and waiting until later. While younger children (between 18 and 24 months) may not meet all the developmental milestones for potty training readiness, such as recognizing their body cues, they tend to be excited and motivated by praise from their caregivers. They're usually potty trained with less resistance than older children. On the other hand, children between 2 and 3 years of age tend to exhibit more developmental readiness, including understanding and recognizing body cues, but may have a healthy need for control and autonomy that makes potty training more difficult.

Research suggests that children who are potty trained too early (before they are developmentally ready) are at higher risk for prolonged training and/or toileting problems. And potty training later than 42 months (3.5 years old) can hinder a child's self-esteem and physiological development (including bladder and bowel control) as they grow older.

Generally speaking, potty training works best when the child is ready to control much of the process, so it tends to be much easier and less stressful for everyone if you wait until your child is ready. After all, children learn best when they are taught something they genuinely want to learn, when they want to learn it. Potty training will go much more smoothly when your child is an eager partner in the process.

Much of the pressure that comes from potty training stems from the notion that there is one specific age at which your child *should* be potty trained. Instead, your child's readiness for potty training will be dependent on your child's unique physiological, motor, cognitive, verbal, and emotional/social development—and *your own readiness.*

You'll want to ensure that your child has reached the necessary milestones before you start potty training. After all, being able to use the bathroom independently involves a complex set of motor, cognitive, verbal, and emotional skills. During this time, your child is learning all about their body and beginning to make the connection between their bodily sensations and appropriate responses. They must also visualize all of the steps involved in the potty process, including the fact that they need to go, and they must develop a plan on how to get to the restroom, sit on the potty and eliminate, and remain on the potty long enough to finish.

In addition, your child will also be using their motor skills to walk to the potty, push down their pants, sit down, stand up, pull their pants up, flush the toilet, and wash their hands. They are also trying to understand your explanations, expectations, instructions, and reactions, while also expressing their own feelings about using the potty. It's a lot to manage all at once, which is why it is a skill that is dependent on preexisting developmental milestones.

Signs That Your Child Is Ready to Start

As noted earlier, you need to be mindful of your child's developmental milestones prior to beginning the potty training process. Keep in mind, though, that your child does not need to demonstrate *all* of these signs in order to signal that they are ready. You can also be proactive by teaching your child some of these skills before starting to set them up for success.

Physiological Development

Before you begin potty training, make sure that your child demonstrates an awareness of the need to eliminate, either by grunting, hiding, squatting, or going rod in the face. Look out for an absence of bowel movements at night, dry diapers for long periods of time (around 2 hours), urinating a lot at one time, and some regularity of bowel movements.

Motor Skills

Your child's ability to walk, handle their clothing (push down and pull up pants, for example), and remain seated long enough to eliminate successfully are all essential skills needed for potty training. Boys typically learn how to pull up their underwear and pants between 29 months and 33 months; girls tend to learn this skill slightly earlier. You can teach your child these skills by demonstrating how to dress and undress, and by making sure their clothing is easy to remove.

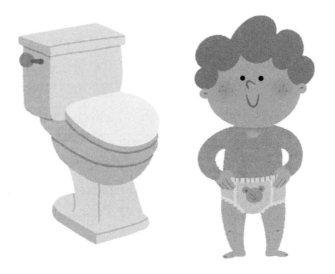

Cognitive and Verbal Skills

Learning to use the toilet independently involves complex cognitive skills. For instance, your child must be able to comprehend the connection between their body sensations that signal needing to eliminate and taking the appropriate action to do so. They also must be able to imagine the potty once they feel the urge to eliminate (which requires symbolic thought), devise a plan on how they will get there (which requires problem-solving skills), stop what they're doing at the moment (which takes impulse control and delayed gratification skills), and hold their plan long enough in their memory to carry it out. They must also resist distraction on the way to the potty (which requires memory and concentration abilities). These skills surface around 12 months and become better established by age 2.

Around age 2, you'll begin to see your child's problem-solving skills over and over again, such as how to get their beloved toy back from their sibling. This is a sign they are cognitively ready for potty training. Your child should be able to follow simple instructions, engage in symbolic play (like using an object to represent something else, such as a banana representing a telephone), and imitate and model behavior. It's important, too, that they have the vocabulary for potty training terms, such as *pee, poop*, and *potty*. Keep in mind that it's not essential that your child can *say* these words. They just need to be able to signal that they need to use the potty through nonverbal language. Having the language down just helps the process go more smoothly. Being able to communicate that they would like their diaper changed is an excellent sign they are ready to be potty trained, as they are demonstrating that they recognize (and dislike) the feeling of being wet and can communicate their needs effectively. It's also beneficial (but not imperative) if your child has the language skills necessary to communicate any problems, confusion, or fears related to potty training.

Emotional and Social Skills

Emotional and social skills are the subtlest of all the developmental milestones. You want to be on the lookout for signs of self-mastery, desire for parental approval, and increased self-reliance. These signs are often manifested in "less than

Common Potty Training Myths

① My child will let me know when they're ready.

Oftentimes, potty training is delayed because parents are waiting for their child to clearly communicate to them that they are ready. While this is the case for some families, most children will not explicitly communicate their readiness. Rather, they will let you know through subtle, indirect signs—like being able to follow simple directions, communicating when they are hungry and thirsty, and reciting their ABCs. These are all indirect cues your child may be ready to potty train.

② Boys are harder to potty train.

While studies show that boys commonly potty train later than girls, it does not mean that boys have a harder time with the process (or that you will either!). And the difference in time is a matter of days or months, not years. In fact, when it comes to potty training, little girls and boys are much more similar than different.

③ You must start potty training by X age.

There is no magic age at which potty training should begin. While children commonly begin the process between 18 and 36 months, remember that every child is different and will start potty training when they're ready.

④ Potty training is really hard.

As a first-time parent, you might assume that this process is going to be super stressful. But it doesn't have to be as complicated or dreadful as you may envision. Minimize the stress by ensuring your child is developmentally ready and you are mentally prepared to embark on this new journey. Keep it as simple as possible and expect (and try to embrace) accidents and regressions.

desirable" behaviors, such as hiding during a bowel movement. However, this is a good sign that your child is more aware of social expectations. Other positive signs include your child imitating the behaviors of others, demonstrating a basic understanding of what the potty is used for, and/or expressing an interest in the potty. Your child may become fascinated with you using the potty, want to help you flush the toilet, or look inside the toilet (and even throw toys in there too). These are all signs your child may be ready to begin potty training.

If your child was born prematurely, has physical or mental difficulties, or has a speech delay or any other developmental delays, they may not be ready to potty train until later than other children. See Chapter 6 for more information about children with special needs.

Who's the Boss? (Hint: You)

While much of the focus is on whether or not your child is developmentally ready for potty training, one of the most crucial components to the success of potty training is whether *you* are ready to embark on this journey. Potty training is a parent-directed activity that depends on your ability to fully commit to the process and maintain consistency. It is normal for parents—especially first-timers—to start and stop training because they're not ready or don't feel equipped to see it through. While this can be confusing for young children, the

HERE ARE COMMON SIGNS YOUR CHILD IS READY TO BEGIN POTTY TRAINING:

Physiological Signs

▶ Remains free of bowel movements overnight
▶ Has regular and predictable bowel movements
▶ Maintains a dry diaper for 2 hours or is dry after naps

Motor Signs

▶ Can walk and sit
▶ Has the ability to push down and pull up pants

Cognitive and Verbal Signs

▶ Demonstrates the need to use the potty through verbal and nonverbal language
▶ Can follow simple directions
▶ Can put toys and other belongings in their right place
▶ Can recite their ABCs or other songs
▶ Lets you know when they've soiled their diaper
▶ Can use potty lingo like *pee, poop,* and *potty*

Emotional and Social Signs

▶ Can sit in one spot for 2 to 5 minutes
▶ Asks to wear underwear or sit on the potty chair
▶ Imitates parental behavior
▶ Shows interest in the toilet
▶ Demonstrates independence and uses the word *no*
▶ Engages in symbolic play
▶ Isn't resistant to learning to use the toilet

start/stop dance can also increase your anxiety and ambivalence. That's why it's crucial to be honest about whether you're ready for this journey. Keep in mind, though, that if your child shows signs of being developmentally ready for potty training, you need to take steps toward mentally preparing yourself for the journey ahead. Try to avoid holding up the process out of your own anxiety and ambivalence.

Remember, your mindset is crucial to the success of this process. Negativity, anxiety, and ambivalence will color your parenting decisions and create unnecessary power struggles between you and your child. It's easy to fixate on all the work or whether you are doing it the right way, but this mindset is counterproductive. Yes, there will be accidents. There might even be setbacks and regressions. But there will also be fun potty dances and bonding time.

Try to enjoy the process, rather than solely focusing on the end result. Even as a first-time parent, you can walk into this process fully trusting in the fact that your child *will* learn to potty train in their own time. Your confidence in them (and yourself) will be the motivation and inspiration they need to persevere. Imagine how amazing it will feel to know you played a critical role in one of your child's first major milestones! Reaching this milestone means they are no longer a baby. Your child will have officially reached a thrilling level of independence. Your excitement in this transition will only add to their success.

It's best to start potty training with a fun, positive spirit that also conveys a sense of confidence and authority. Keep things simple and avoid comparing your journey with that of other parents. And rest assured that you will walk away from this experience with a better understanding of your child and their unique learning style.

Looking Back and Moving Forward
Let's recap the major points of this chapter:

▶ There is no magical age at which potty training should begin. While most children will be ready to begin between 18 and 36 months, every child is different regarding when they are ready and how long it will take them to master this skill.

▶ Prior to starting the process, make sure your child is developmentally ready by being aware of physiological, motor, cognitive, speech, and social/emotional developmental milestones.

▶ Your child will probably not tell you when they are ready to begin potty training. Instead, watch for subtle, indirect signs that convey readiness.

▶ Learning to potty train is a major transition for your child. Your positive attitude and confidence in them (and yourself) will keep them motivated and inspired throughout this process of ups and downs.

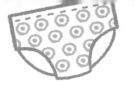
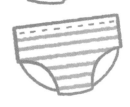

CHAPTER 2

Preparing for the Big Event

AS WITH ANY TRANSITION, potty training works best if you think it through before you start. Here's where you'll find the equipment and supplies you need, how to prepare your child for the process, and a quick run through of what to expect as you enter this uncharted territory.

How to Prepare Yourself

Since you've never guided someone through this process before, it's important to become mentally prepared to begin the potty training journey. Mental preparedness begins with committing to have a positive and confident attitude for yourself and your child, setting aside time to begin the process, gradually introducing your child to the idea, and gathering the supplies you will need.

This program entails 3 days of intensive potty training at

home and brief public outings. You will begin by having your child run around your home commando (without any diapers or underwear on) and then slowly introduce underwear after several successful eliminations on the potty. The first few days will require your undivided attention and commitment to learning your child's potty cues and cleaning up accidents.

For busy parents, 3 days can seem like a big commitment. The idea of being stuck inside for several days with a busy child may not seem like fun, but this is essential to the success of potty training. During these days, you will learn how to read your child's unique potty cues and they will learn to associate their bodily sensations with running to the bathroom. So set aside the time when you won't be distracted by work or other commitments. Block off these days on the calendar so that nothing else gets in the way during that time. This is a big learning curve for both of you.

> **Set aside the time when you won't be distracted by work or other commitments.**

In addition, remember to talk to your partner and other primary caregivers so that you're on the same page about beginning the potty training process. You might also want to consult with your child's day-care provider, preschool teacher, babysitter, and anyone else who will be expected to offer support during this journey.

It's also important to note that you shouldn't start potty training when your child is sick or dealing with a major life transition like a new school, a parent's new work schedule, or around the due date of a new sibling.

How to Prepare Your Child

Prior to beginning the process, you'll need to mentally prepare your child by getting them acquainted with their new potty, teaching them how to dress and undress themselves, showing them how to wash their hands, and teaching them the new potty lingo.

Make Time for Daily Play and Connection

Potty training is a big transition for everyone, and it may create some stress for your child. Imagine you're starting a new job. Although you're excited, you'll probably have some nervous anticipation since there are several unknowns, like new coworkers and procedures. This is the same for your child when it comes to potty training. Help lessen your child's anxiety by loading up on snuggles and playtime prior to and during this transition. Try to dedicate at least 10 minutes per day to one-on-one playtime to give your child extra TLC during this big change. This will go a long way in reducing behavioral issues as your child is more likely to feel connected with you and less anxious about the change ahead.

Invite Them to the Restroom with You

Introduce your child to the toilet by inviting them into the bathroom when you go. Keep in mind that children tend to identify more with same-sex caregivers when it comes to potty training, so it's optimal if, for instance, dads (or other male relatives) take their sons to the restroom to model how to use the toilet. You can say things like, "I drank a lot of water, and now I have the potty feeling. It's time to put my pee in the potty." Once you're on the toilet, you can say something like, "Wow, here it comes! Do you hear that sound? Pee goes in the potty." Encourage them by letting them know it will be their turn soon. You can say something like, "Pretty soon you will go pee in the potty just like me! How exciting!" Potty trips are also an excellent opportunity to encourage your child to become involved in the process by allowing them to flush the toilet and say, "Bye-bye, pee (or poop)!" This helps them learn how to flush the toilet, allows them to see where pee and poop should go, and gets them used to the new potty lingo.

Introduce Their New Potty

When introducing your child to their potty chair, avoid making it seem like it's a new toy. Keep the potty chair strictly for business and bring your child to it after diaper changes. Together, you can put it in a place where your child frequently plays. In the early days of training, you'll want to have the potty close by so your child can get to it quickly when they feel the urge to go.

Practice the Dressing/Undressing Routine

Begin dressing your child in clothing that is conducive to potty training. For instance, buy pants that are easy to push down and pull up (avoid overalls and pants with tricky buttons) and begin practicing this task with your child as early as possible. You can start by having your child push down their pants and pull them back up during diaper changes.

Bridge the Gap between Diapers and the Potty

If possible, start changing your child's diapers near their potty, as this subtly reinforces the connection between the two. Also, after your child has a poopy diaper, invite them to join you as you flush the contents down the toilet. This helps them learn that the appropriate place for poop is in the potty. This also helps them learn the ritual of flushing and saying "bye-bye" to poop and pee.

Read Books to Start the Potty Conversation

Books are an excellent way to introduce your child to the concept of potty training. They help spark a conversation about the topic that is fun and nonthreatening. They also reinforce the idea that going potty is a normal, universal part of daily life for everyone—even animals. If you have pets, this is a great opportunity to discuss how they go potty and what the rules are for them (like going outside or using a litter box).

Reading books about anatomy will also help your child learn about and give words to what is happening in their body. This will help them learn to associate their body signals with their need to go to the potty. Give those signals a name (like "potty feeling"), and teach them that everyone experiences these sensations.

Don't Underestimate the Power of Play

Play is an excellent tool for teaching your child about potty training. While you're preparing your child to begin, initiate lots of pretend play in which you both teach a doll, a stuffed animal, or an action figure how to use the potty. If you sense that your child is anxious or resistant to potty training, use play to model how to work around those issues. For instance, if the doll is afraid of the potty, reassure the doll that the potty is safe and fun. Let the doll know it's okay to feel scared to try new things, but show that these experiences can be fun and rewarding. Show the doll being brave and trying new things after a little reassurance.

This is also a great opportunity to model a positive attitude about accidents. You can reassure the doll by saying, "I know it's hard to get to the potty sometimes. I'll help you clean up, and we can try again next time." Avoid conveying too much acceptance of accidents during role-playing by saying things like "It's okay," because, well, it's not. Instead, encourage the doll to keep a positive attitude and keep trying, and let the

Potty Language to Avoid

Avoid using negative language like *stinky poop* and *yucky pee*. You never want to refer to your child's diaper as "smelly" or "gross," as this can contribute to your child's resistance, apprehension, and discomfort around potty training. You want to convey to your child that using the toilet is a natural thing that all humans do. Normalize this process, and try not to create negative connotations about going to the potty.

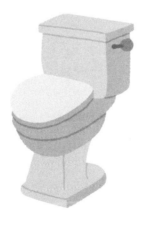

doll know you're with them every step of the way. You'll want to convey understanding and compassion while avoiding the message that it's fine to have accidents. Play is also a wonderful way for you to practice your potty training script.

What to Buy

Since this is your first time potty training, you probably need some guidance on getting the right supplies to get started. You'll want to involve your child as much as possible. Remember, young children yearn for a sense of control and autonomy, so you'll want to provide them with lots of opportunities to make decisions during this time. Also, keep in mind that this process should begin weeks before you begin potty training so that you and your child have plenty of time to prepare, both mentally and practically, for the journey ahead. Here are the supplies you'll need.

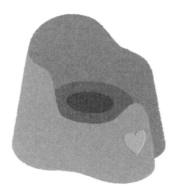

POTTY CHAIR

Chair or Seat?

When it comes to the choice between a potty chair or a potty training seat, you might have to try out both and see which your child prefers. Here are the pros and cons of each.

Potty chairs are often appealing to young children because they sport fun colors, entertaining sounds, and their favorite characters. They are usually much less intimidating for young children due to their small size. They are also easy to sit on and do not leave the child's feet dangling. (Children can have difficulty controlling their voiding muscles when their feet are dangling.) Potty chairs are easy to place around your home for quick access. When shopping for one, make sure to select a chair that is portable and easy to clean. Steer clear

Ideally, the potty chair will be easy to access to ensure success.

of potty chairs that come with splash guards if you have a boy because they can hurt themselves as they sit down.

Where should you put your potty chair? Leave it where your child frequently plays. Ideally, the potty chair will be easy to access to ensure success. Buy a chair for each floor of your house.

The downsides of potty chairs are that they can be difficult to clean (particularly poop), and they are often not available in public places like preschools and restaurants. Furthermore, they can take up space in the bathroom and other parts of your home.

As an alternative, your child can use a potty training seat that sits on any toilet seat. Your child will be less likely to be afraid of going potty in public if they are used to using

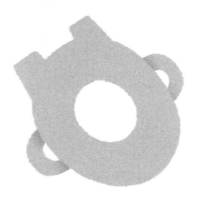

POTTY TRAINING SEAT

a toilet at home. And potty seats involve significantly less cleanup than potty chairs.

The downside of potty training seats, however, is that they can be intimidating because of how large they are. Young children may fear they will fall into the toilet. The splash and other sounds can also be a deterrent for little ones. Potty training seats also can't be used in areas without toilets, such as parks.

If you decide to go with a potty training seat, purchase a step stool so that your child's feet won't dangle. Their feet should rest on a flat surface when they're using the toilet.

Children younger than 30 months generally prefer a potty chair. Children over 30 months are usually okay with

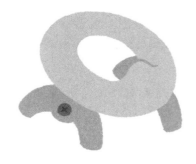

TRAVEL POTTY CHAIR

a potty training seat on an adult toilet. A little trial and error might be necessary as you learn which your child is most comfortable with. Most parents eventually purchase a potty training seat once their child is older and fully potty trained.

You will also want to purchase a travel potty chair or training seat for when you're in public. There are also travel potties that can be used as a potty chair and a potty training seat.

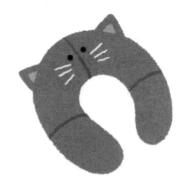

TRAVEL POTTY TRAINING SEAT

Extra Underwear

While underwear won't come into play until after the first couple of days, you'll want to stock up on lots of extra pairs now. Get your child involved in picking out their underwear by letting them choose their favorite characters and purchasing two to three bags of new, fun underwear. You'll be able to encourage your child to keep their favorite characters dry and comfortable.

Easy-On-and-Off Pants

As your child begins the potty training process, you'll want to stick with easy-on-and-off pants. Avoid rompers and overalls. You'll also want to steer clear of pants with zippers, buttons, and drawstrings because they're harder for your child to manage. Instead, buy pants and shorts with elastic waists that are simple to remove since your child will be learning the sensation of needing to go and will have lots of close calls. Also, the goal is to teach your child to be as self-sufficient as possible, so clothing that is simple for them to manage is essential.

Rewards

Depending on your personal preference, you may want to purchase small treats, like M&M's, to give your child when they use the potty. Some parents prefer sticker charts or small toys, while others would rather offer simple verbal praise to reward the behavior. (See Chapter 3 for more about positive reinforcement and rewards.)

Flushable Wipes

Stock up on flushable wipes since a fast transition from baby wipes to toilet paper can be uncomfortable for your child. Flushable wipes are much softer than toilet paper and more familiar to your child. However, some children won't mind using toilet paper, so use your discretion on this one.

Cleaning Supplies

Prepare for accidents by having cleaning supplies stocked and ready to go. You will want disinfectant spray, wipes, and paper towels for the inevitable cleanups.

Step Stool

A small wooden or plastic step stool will help your child get up on the potty training seat and sit comfortably. It will also give your child a sense of safety and stability while they are high up on the toilet. Your little one will also need a step stool to reach the sink to wash their hands. Some potty chairs convert to a stool to cut down on bathroom clutter.

Exclusive Potty Activities

You'll want to keep a basket near the potty chair or toilet (if you're using a training seat) filled with books, a coloring pad, a magnetic drawing board, and water-reveal coloring books. You can also include toys and trinkets your child might enjoy. Be sure these items are used only for potty time to keep them exciting and fun.

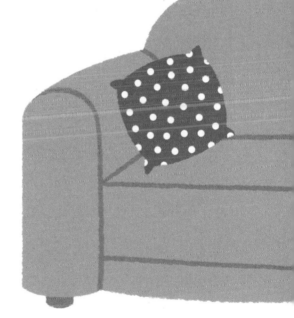

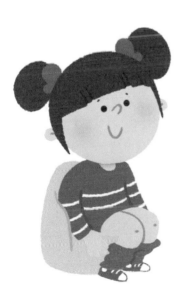

Car Seat and Stroller Protector Pads

Protector pads are a great way to protect your car seat and stroller and relieve some of the stress of going on public outings while still potty training. Bonus: These pads are machine washable!

New Toys and Activities

In addition to the activities to be used during potty time, you may want to buy a few new items for you and your child to do while you remain indoors for the first few days. Play-Doh sets, coloring books, and puzzles can help keep your little one entertained during that time.

Simple and Easy Snacks and Meals

During the first few days, your attention will primarily be on watching your child like a hawk. There will be little time to cook, so stock up on simple and easy snacks and meals for those first few days.

Other Things to Consider

Now that you know the must-haves to get you started, there are a few other items you also might want—as well as tasks to get out of the way—before you begin potty training.

Floor and Furniture Protection

Since accidents are often unavoidable during potty training, you may want to roll up rugs and place towels on sofas and chairs.

Are You Ready for the Big Event?

You need to have all your ducks in a row before you start potty training. Go through this checklist to make sure you're ready:

- [ ] You have all the necessary supplies handy and ready to go.

- [ ] You have begun preparing your child for the process by reading books on potty training, having them pick out their underwear, and letting them know the process will be starting soon.

- [ ] You have scheduled a date to begin potty training and have set aside other major responsibilities during this time period.

- [ ] You have made other family members aware of the plan.

- [ ] You know this is a process and not a single event. You are prepared for the ups and downs of potty training, including accidents and other setbacks.

Toilet Targets

Many parents prefer to start their boys off in the sitting position. (See Chapter 4 for more on this.) If you decide to teach your son to urinate while standing, he may enjoy having toilet targets like Cheerios so that he has something to aim for when going potty. You can also use food coloring so that your child can see what color the water turns when their pee makes it into the toilet!

Looking Back and Moving Forward

Let's recap the major points of this chapter:

▶ You need to be mentally and practically prepared for the big event.

▶ Ideally, the potty training process should begin *before* the big event. Introduce your child to the idea of potty training through books, play, inviting them to the bathroom with you, and other strategies.

▶ Make sure your home is prepared for the big event by purchasing a potty chair or potty training seat, a travel potty, underwear, easy-on-and-off clothing, rewards, cleaning supplies, exclusive potty activities, and more.

▶ Since you'll be stuck inside for the first few days, consider keeping meals and snacks simple and purchasing new activities to entertain your child.

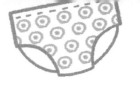
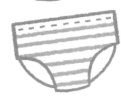

CHAPTER 3

Ground Rules

SINCE YOU'RE THE BOSS, you get to set the rules for your child, but as a first-timer, you might not realize that there are a few you must follow too. Here's what you both need to know.

Bathroom Talk (Choose Your Terms)

Before you start potty training, you need to decide what language you are going to use, since you'll be teaching this lingo to your child. Your language throughout is critical. It helps your child communicate with you and colors their perception of their bodies and the potty process. Whether you use clinically correct terms like *urine* and *bowel movement* or more informal terms like *poop* and *pee* is up to you. Just stay consistent, and steer clear of words you don't want your child to pick up and terms that carry a negative connotation. It's also ideal if the words are easy for your child to pronounce.

Common words for urination include *pee, pee-pee, wee, wee-wee, tinkle,* and *number one.* Feces is often referred to as *poop, poopie, doo-doo, ka-ka,* and *number two.* There are also several terms for the room where the toilet is located, including *bathroom, restroom, little boy's* (or *little girl's*) *room,* and many more.

For anatomy-related terms, you can teach your son that he has a *penis.* Your daughter can be told that she has a *vagina* and that urine comes out in front of her vagina and in front of where the poop comes out. This understanding will come in handy when she is learning how to wipe from front to back so that she doesn't transfer poop into her vagina.

Find out what terms caregivers, like day-care staff, babysitters, and family members, use. While it's best if every caregiver uses the same lingo to avoid confusing your child, it's okay if they use different terms—as long as your child is comfortable using those words.

What to Say

While choosing potty lingo before starting the potty training process is important, it's also essential to be intentional about the overall language you want to use throughout the journey.

Remember, your child is in complete control regarding whether they use the potty. Your role is to empower and appeal to their desire for independence without starting a power struggle or causing feelings of shame or failure. The language you use, and your overall demeanor, will mean the difference between a battle and a partnership. Here are some recommendations on what to say to make the process easier for both you and your child.

"It's time to go potty."

While your child decides whether they will use the potty, it's up to you to provide the structure. Your child is likely to respond with a simple no if you ask them, "Do you need to go potty?" Instead, set yourself up for success by telling them that it's time to sit on the potty.

"Would you like to go potty in two minutes or five minutes?"

Young children have a healthy need for control and independence. Avoid power struggles by giving your child choices about when they go potty. Pick two choices you are equally fine with (2 minutes or 5 minutes, for example), and then allow them to choose. You can also let your child choose if they want to go on the big potty (the toilet) or the little potty (the potty chair). Giving your child a sense of control over when and where they potty can be extremely empowering.

"We're about to eat dinner. Let's go potty before we eat."

Transitions are your friend when potty training. Teach your child to sit on the potty before and after transitions early on. Prepare them for upcoming transitions by giving them a heads-up about what's happening next and then tell them to sit on the potty first. This is a great way to prevent accidents and create a sense of routine around the process. You can also use *when/then* statements to communicate what you want and what your child can expect after potty time. For instance, "When you sit on the potty, then we can go play at the park!"

"Be sure to go to the potty when you get the potty feeling."

Help your child recognize their body's cues by giving them a simple reminder to sit on the potty when they need to go. Have a discussion with your child about bodily sensations associated with needing to go. For instance, people often pass gas prior to a bowel movement. If you notice this, help your child associate the smell of gas with the need to poop and encourage them to sit on the potty. Recognizing your child's cues (such as the "potty dance") and pointing out the cues in the moment is also a great way to teach your child how to associate bodily sensations with the need to go.

"Be sure to keep your underwear (or character) dry. They like feeling dry and comfortable."

When your child starts to wear underwear, you can encourage them to keep their favorite characters dry and comfortable. This will help empower your child and give them a sense of autonomy and control if they feel they're responsible for taking care of their favorite characters.

"I'm so proud of you for keeping (character on underwear) dry!"

Shower your child with praise during this process. Be as specific as possible when you compliment your child so that they can learn exactly what behaviors are appropriate and encouraged. Positive reinforcement is a great way to help your child draw the connection between holding their pee for the potty and keeping their body (and underwear) dry.

When praising your child, focus on their effort and hard work (for example, "I see all the hard work you're doing to keep your underwear dry! Fantastic effort!") rather than making vague global statements like, "You're a good kid!" Global statements can lead to a sense of failure when your child has an accident, while praising hard work encourages your child to keep trying when there is a setback.

When it comes to praise, don't overdo it or appear too emotionally invested, which can create pressure for your child and take their control away. Instead, praise your child for their successes but keep it short and sweet.

"You're such a big kid. You're going potty just like I do!"

As stated above, young children tend to have a healthy need for independence and control. Praising them for being a "big kid" is a great way to appeal to their desire for greater autonomy. Your child also loves imitating you, so acknowledging the ways in which they are behaving just like you can be extremely encouraging. Keep in mind, however, that this form of praise might not work for every child. Some children become anxious being told they are a big kid because they want to continue being treated like a baby. As with any tip in this book, always keep your unique child in mind.

"Let me know when you have to go potty."

As your child becomes more aware of their bodily cues and sensations and begins to initiate potty time, start telling them to let you know when they need to go, especially when out in public. This again empowers your child and encourages greater potty independence.

What Not to Say

Try not to show disappointment if your child sits on the potty but doesn't go. Instead, praise their effort ("Thanks for trying!") and make a plan to try again ("We can try again after lunch").

Avoid punishing and criticizing your child when they have accidents. Saying things like, "Eww, that's yucky. You pooped in your underwear. Now (character) is all dirty and smelly!" only creates a sense of failure, shame, and doubt. The early years are a crucial time in the development of a healthy self-concept. Your comments will either work toward supporting your child's budding sense of autonomy or fill your child with self-doubt and low self-esteem.

> **Avoid punishing and criticizing your child when they have accidents.**

If potty training becomes anxiety-provoking and a power struggle, your child may feel shame and may doubt their ability to succeed. This self-doubt will likely interfere with their effort to attain autonomy and impede your child's success. On the other hand, your child is more likely to develop self-esteem and a sense of independence if they feel supported.

Patience, Patience, and More Patience

Just saying the words *potty training* can evoke mixed emotions. This process takes so much patience. It is a huge developmental milestone for your child, and they may take a while to fully learn it. Potty training is also a huge, sometimes overwhelming, parenting milestone—especially for a parent who has never been through it before. It's common to feel flustered and frustrated, especially in the early stages, so having patience with yourself is important.

Your mindset walking into this process is critical! What you say to yourself about *your ability* to successfully teach your child this new skill and your perception of *your child's ability* to learn it are crucial to the success of this journey. Remember that potty training is a unique journey for *everyone*. It's not a race. Your child doesn't have to be done with potty training by a particular date. You haven't failed if potty training takes you longer than it took your friends and family. Try to focus on the process rather than the end result. You'll discover more patience and might even be surprised at how fast it goes. Why not enjoy it? Trust the process. You got this.

Another thing about patience: Your child knows when you have little of it. They are incredibly intuitive and can detect impatience before you even open your mouth. Remember, early childhood is all about gaining control over the environment. When your child senses that you are frustrated with them and are trying to control the process, they may become resistant in an effort to regain control. And when your child senses your impatience, they internalize it. It is very difficult for children to learn under stress.

So when you see your child becoming stressed and resisting potty training, it might be a good time to ask yourself, *How do I feel about this process? What are my intentions and expectations? Have I placed my child on an unrealistic deadline?* and *Am I approaching this process with tension and stress or trust and positivity?* These questions will help you reevaluate your expectations and adjust your thoughts and beliefs about the process. Remember, you set the emotional tone. Your child is following your lead; if you feel stressed and impatient with the process, they will too.

What About Rewards?

Positive reinforcement can be powerful for the learning process. This involves adding something like verbal praise or a small treat whenever your child exhibits a desired behavior, such as using the potty. An example of positive reinforcement is rewards. Rewards come in handy when reinforcing any new skill, and they're especially helpful in potty training. Giving a reward directly after the desired behavior (for example, going pee on the potty) increases the likelihood of seeing that behavior again because it lets your child know in a very clear way that they are on the right track. Make sure the reward comes *immediately* after the desired behavior. This means promising your child their favorite dessert for lunch after they go potty in the morning will not be effective. Also, rewards must be short-term: giving TV time as a reward is not recommended because it's too long in duration. If your child can hold on to the reward for longer than 30 seconds, then it's too long.

> **Make sure the reward comes *immediately* after the desired behavior.**

Positive reinforcement can take the shape of verbal and nonverbal praise (clapping, smiles, hugs), treats, toys, sticker charts, or anything else that is reinforcing to your child. When it comes to verbal praise, saying things like, "Yay! You went potty!" and "I'm happy you're keeping your pants dry!" work well because they are descriptive, letting your child know exactly what they are doing right and what you expect. Verbal praise also increases their self-esteem and motivation.

However, avoid excessing praising, as it can inadvertently cause your child to feel pressured to perform well and never make mistakes. Instead, focus on their determination and how hard they are working and how much you love them (despite their accidents), and let them know you have confidence they will succeed. Also, when deciding how to praise your child, keep their unique personality in mind. While one child might love being called a big kid, for instance, this might cause another child anxiety. Also, pick and choose what praises come naturally for you. You always want to be sure your praises are authentic because your child will be able to sense when they're not.

Here's a quick list of verbal praise to get you started:

- I love how you went potty all by yourself. Wow!
- Look at you keeping your pants dry! What a big kid!
- Yay! You told me when you needed to go potty. Well done!
- What a big kid you are, wiping and flushing all on your own. I'm proud of you.
- You're doing great on your own, but if you need help, just let me know!
- You are working so hard and making such great progress!
- I'm so proud of you for all your hard work.
- It's so exciting seeing you go potty all by yourself!
- Thank you for helping me clean up your accident.
- Thanks for letting me know you had an accident. You are working so hard to learn to go potty. Let's clean you up and try again.

Positive reinforcement may need to be a gradual process. For instance, if your child is disinterested in or resistant to even sitting on the potty, you may have to start rewarding them for standing by the potty, sitting on the potty with their clothes on, and then sitting on the potty without their pants on. Once your child is comfortable sitting on the potty, you may begin rewarding for successes in the potty, and then eventually for keeping their underwear dry for extended periods of time. Each child will begin this process in a different place. Follow your child's lead and reward small steps. Quickly move to the next level once your child has mastered a particular level. For instance, once your child has mastered pulling down their pants and sitting on the potty, move on to rewarding successful potty trips.

Each child will begin this process in a different place.

You may also want to buy small treats—like M&M's, chocolate-covered raisins, SweeTARTS, gummy bears, potato chips, or pretzels—as rewards. You may decide to keep the treats in a clear jar in the restroom for your child to see. You can give your child one small treat (one M&M, for example) for going pee and two for poop. If you are not a fan of treats, you can give your child a small toy, but keep in mind that your child will have numerous eliminations throughout the first few days. Some parents let their child play with a new toy and then once they're done, return it to the toy basket for them to

Establish a Potty Routine

Establishing a potty routine early on helps make going potty a normal part of the day. It eliminates the stress of needing to remind your child about it every 30 to 60 minutes and makes power struggles less likely. You can help them remember the routine by creating a potty training chart that has visuals of the common times during the day that your child will go to the potty.

Great times include the following:

- First thing in the morning

- Before and after meals

- Before playtime and screen time

- Right before and after outings

- When you arrive at public places, like stores, day care, and school

- Before and after naps

- Before bath time

- Right before bedtime

pick again later. You could also save toys for more advanced accomplishments like accident-free days.

Another option is to use a sticker chart. Have your child place one sticker on the chart when they pee and two when they poop. You can use this in conjunction with the small treats and toys for added incentive. Sticker charts are a nice visual way to show your child how successful they are.

Keep in mind that you will want to gradually eliminate the sticker chart as most children will lose interest in it around day 3. To do this, simply don't remind your child about their sticker after potty successes and then eventually take the chart down. You will also want to gradually take away the small treat. Wait until your child is consistently using the potty for a week or two before slowly withdrawing the treats. For instance, over time you may decide to give your child a treat only when they poop, then only when they initiate going potty without prompting, and then only when they have no accidents in a day (and then several days). You may also consider increasing the reward based on the accomplishment. For instance, a good potty day with no accidents can mean a special dessert.

Food and Drink

What goes in must come out! During the early days of training, you'll want to load your child up with lots of liquids in

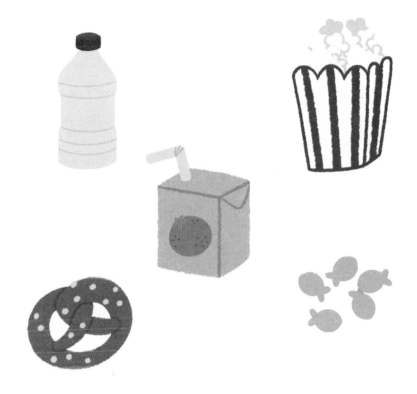

order to give them plenty of opportunities to practice going potty. You can give them water and/or watered-down juice to make sure they get their fair share of liquids. But do not give them excessive amounts of juice or they can get diarrhea. Diluting the juice is your safest bet. You'll also want to offer them lots of foods that are hydrating, as well as salty snacks to make them thirsty. Offer them a high-fiber diet with lots of fruits, vegetables, and whole grains to help prevent constipation. (See Chapter 9 for more on constipation and diarrhea.)

Recommended drinks and hydrating foods include the following:

- Water
- Milk
- Watered-down juice
- Decaffeinated tea
- Coconut water
- Smoothies
- Popsicles
- Watery fruits like watermelon and grapes (just be sure to cut these up into small pieces)

Recommended snacks include the following:

- Chips
- Crackers
- Goldfish
- Popcorn
- Fruit with peanut butter
- Pretzels

Clothing vs. Clothing Optional

In the early days of potty training, you'll want your child to be naked from the waist down. (See Chapter 4 for more information.) Over time, you'll introduce stretchy, loose-fitting pants with no buttons or zippers that are easy to take off and put on. If the weather is warm, you can opt for shorts or skirts. In the winter, you can put on sweatpants or leggings as long as they can easily be taken off.

Looking Back and Moving Forward
Let's recap the major points of this chapter:

▶ When it comes to your bathroom talk, keep potty training lingo short and consistent. Make sure these words are easy for your child to pronounce, and avoid using words you don't want your child to pick up.

▶ Be intentional about the language you use during potty training. Keep your words and tone positive, instructional, and empowering. Avoid criticizing your child for accidents and potty refusal, as this can create a power struggle and a sense of failure and shame.

▶ Think of potty training as a process and not a one-time event. This mindset will grant you the necessary patience you will need throughout this journey.

▶ Rewards are a form of positive reinforcement and can be effective during the process. They are *not essential* but sure do help. If you decide to give rewards, keep them small and make sure you give them consistently and immediately after the desired behavior.

▶ Establish a potty routine early on to help your child learn that going potty is a normal part of their day. This also helps them learn how to initiate going potty and avoids power struggles.

▶ During the initial days of potty training, load your child up on lots of liquids, watery foods, and salty snacks for lots of opportunities to practice going to the potty.

▶ Have your child wear clothing that is easy to take off and on during the early days of potty training. Avoid clothes with buttons and zippers and try to stick with loose-fitting pants and/or shorts and skirts.

The
Big
Event

You should feel confident that you can help your child successfully use the toilet, but as a first-time parent, you need the knowledge and maybe a bit of guidance and hand-holding to do so. This part gives you both.

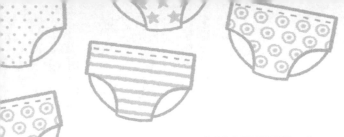

CHAPTER 4

Let's Go Potty!

IT'S TIME TO START! Here's everything you need to know about pee, poop, and accidents.

The Pee and Poop Program

This program is designed to keep potty training as simple and straightforward as possible. Since every family is different, use these steps as general guidelines and tweak the program as you see fit. There will be some trial and error as you learn about your preferred teaching style, your child's unique learning style, and what motivates and frustrates them. Set the emotional tone for the process by staying calm and patient with your child. Follow your child's lead and empower them to listen to their own bodies. Be their cheerleader, encouraging them every step of the way.

Core Principles of the Program

Since you will be tweaking the program to make the potty training process work for your child and your family, here are some core principles to keep in mind as you begin.

Be Positive

As you've already read, children learn best in a relaxed, positive environment with minimal pressure and stress. Always strive to create a partnership with your child. By doing so, you honor that they are in complete control of their bodies, while being fully mindful of your role to motivate and empower them toward greater independence.

Be Clear and Consistent

Throughout the journey, you will want to be clear and consistent with your child. Although this is uncharted territory for both of you, you need to convey a sense of confidence through consistency in your expectations and in your routine, including when and where to potty and the sequence of tasks that occur afterward (wiping, flushing, pulling up underwear and pants, and washing and drying hands).

Be Attentive

Your child will need your undivided attention in the early days of potty training. You will be learning about your child's potty habits and will need to be able to anticipate their needs from hour to hour. Consider keeping a notepad handy to record when your child goes pee and poop. This will help you know the best times to prompt them to use the potty. Fair warning: This attentiveness can be exhausting; try to involve another caregiver in the process so that you can take breaks.

Enjoy the Process

It might seem difficult, but you should focus on enjoying the process and set aside the end result. Try your best to focus on the present moment and lose your expectations of how potty training should go and how long it should take. Your child will learn to use the potty sooner or later. For now, enjoy the fun, silly, and messy moments, knowing full well your child will never be this small again.

Getting Ready

A first-time parent might think that once you get your supplies, it's time to start potty training. But the truth is that you need to take care of more than just the basics before you start this important journey with your child.

Prepare Your Child for the Big Event

Preparing your child for potty training will ideally come weeks before the actual big event. Set them up for success by involving them in the process of picking out their potty gear (including potty chair and underwear), reading books to start the potty conversation, inviting them to accompany you to the bathroom, teaching them to undress and dress themselves independently, and using play to model the potty process and troubleshoot any fears or concerns that may come up.

Pick a Weekend and Stick to It

To jump-start the process, pick a weekend (ideally a long weekend of at least 3 days) where you can fully dedicate your time and attention to potty training. The first days will require you to stay close to home and focus all your energy and attention on your child, so pick a weekend where your schedule is clear. Also, remember that you shouldn't start potty training when your child is sick or dealing with a major life transition.

Day 1: Step-by-Step

The first day of the program is probably the most important because it sets the stage for the days to come. Once you are fully prepared, try to walk into Day 1 with confidence and excitement. You got this!

Step 1: Have a "Goodbye" Ceremony

On the morning of the first day, you will want to hold a fun ceremony where you (and other caregivers involved) and your child formally say goodbye to diapers. Tell your child first thing in the morning that today is the day they become a big kid once and for all and say goodbye to diapers. You can say something like, "Today we are saying bye-bye to diapers. You are a big kid now. Pee and poop go in the toilet from now on. Yay! You are going to go to the potty just like me! When you go pee on the potty, you will get one treat and one sticker to put on your chart. When you poop, you will get two treats and two stickers. Let me know when you get the potty feeling so that I can help you go to the potty."

Start by removing your child's diaper and saying goodbye to that one first. Then go around your home with your child and put all the remaining diapers in a bag or other container. Explain that the diapers will be donated to babies who need them.

Step 2: Go Naked from the Waist Down

You'll want your child to be naked from the waist down at first. You can dress them in a long shirt or dress. This is important for several reasons. First, underwear and pull-ups can resemble diapers because they are warm and fitting. This will only confuse your child and increase the likelihood of accidents. Second, being naked is a great way to teach your child how uncomfortable it is to have an accident because they'll have direct feedback on their skin. Third, you'll want your child to be able to get to the potty quickly in the early days. Extra clothes and underwear only interfere with this. Lastly, you're more likely to see exactly when your child is having an accident if they do not have any underwear or clothes on.

Step 3: Orient Your Child to the Process

After you have the diaper ceremony and remove your child's diaper and pants, let your child know where all the potty chairs (if you're using them) or toilets are and what they need to do if they get the potty feeling. Remind them of what the characters in their potty books did when they got the potty feeling (they sat on the potty). You can even role-play with their doll how to go potty. This all sets the stage for the days and weeks to come, so be as positive and matter of-fact as possible. Create a partnership from the beginning and focus on uplifting and empowering your child.

Step 4: Load up on Liquids and Salty Snacks

After the diaper ceremony and introduction to potty training, start loading up your child on liquids, watery fruits, and salty snacks. You want them to have as many opportunities to practice going potty as possible, especially while you are in the comfort of your home.

Step 5: Watch Your Child and Stay Close to the Potty

Once your child is loaded up with liquids, it's time to watch them like a hawk. Your child will need your full and undivided attention during this process. During these early days, you'll need to become aware of your child's potty habits and try to anticipate their needs from hour to hour. Catching their accidents in progress is essential. Avoid getting distracted by electronics and try to delegate chores and tasks to other caregivers. Since this can be exhausting, try to get other caregivers involved in the process so you can get an occasional break. Keep the potty chair close by (or stay close to the bathroom if you're using a potty training seat).

So how do you know if your child needs to go potty? Some common signs are clutching themselves, jumping up and down in place (also known as the pee-pee dance), fidgeting, restlessness, crossing their legs, and passing gas prior to pooping. If they show these signs, calmly say, "It looks like your pee or poop is coming. Let's go sit on the potty." On average, children will urinate anywhere from 3 to 11 times per day and young children usually need to go to the bathroom within an hour of having a large drink.

Step 6: Prompt and Give Reminders

During the first days of potty training, give your child short prompts and simple reminders to encourage them to sit on the potty. You can say something as simple as "All right, it's time to practice going potty," and calmly and matter-of-factly take them to the potty chair or toilet. Start reminding them every 20 to 30 minutes, and gradually increase the time between prompts after several successful eliminations on the potty with your prompting. The ultimate goal is for your child to respond to the urge to use the potty on their own, without prompts.

Be sure you don't come across as nagging or forceful in your reminders. Avoid saying things like, "Do you have to go potty?" over and over again. Not only is this annoying and frustrating, but the answer will likely be no. Use their cues and the clock to determine when to prompt them, but avoid overprompting to minimize the risk of power struggles.

As they get the hang of it, start to use natural transitions as a way to encourage your child to use the potty. For instance, if you're about to start a new activity, say something like, "I can't wait to play with you! When you go potty, then we can get started." If it's been 45 to 60 minutes since your child's last elimination, or you notice them showing cues, simply take them to the potty and say, "It's time to go potty!" Be fun and lighthearted in your tone and never force your child to sit on the toilet against their will. Encourage them to sit for a minute or two but don't force them to stay on the potty or to actually go potty before they can get up. If they insist that they don't have to go, accept it and try again later.

HERE ARE SOME HELPFUL PROMPTS AND REMINDERS:

▶ Let me know when you need to go potty.

▶ Let me know when you get that potty feeling.

▶ Be sure to keep dry.

▶ It's time to go potty.

▶ When you go potty, then we can have a snack/ treat/play/go to the park.

▶ You're such a big kid going pee on the potty!

▶ I love how you're using the potty like a big kid.

▶ Thanks for trying to go potty! I see you don't have to go yet, so let's try again soon.

Step 7: Reward with Simple Praise

Once your child has had a successful elimination in the potty, praise them with a simple, "You went pee in the potty. Yes, pee goes in the potty. Way to go!" To keep your language positive, avoid pointing out where it doesn't go (on the floor or in clothing) and just stick with where it *does* go. Keep this short, simple, and matter-of-fact. While tangible rewards, like a small treat, toy, or sticker, are optional, the American Academy of Pediatrics recommends the use of incentives to encourage your child to learn the necessary potty skills and maintain motivation to keep trying. Just be sure the reward is not so big that it distracts them from the act itself. For instance, one M&M or gummy bear will suffice for a successful urine elimination in the potty. Remember, with any positive reinforcement (whether it's verbal praise or a small reward), be sure to give it immediately after the desired behavior.

Day 2: Step-by-Step

Day 2 will not be much different from Day 1 in terms of technique. The biggest new event on Day 2 is one public outing, if you and your child are ready.

Step 1: Stay Naked

Your child is still learning how to understand their body cues, and you are still learning about their potty habits. Keep your child naked from the waist down while at home on Day 2.

Step 2: Continue the Liquids and Salty Snacks

Continue to give your child ample amounts of liquids, watery fruits, and salty snacks to give them plenty of opportunities to practice going to the potty.

Step 3: Build Potty Time into the Daily Routine

Now is a great time to begin making potty time a part of your daily routine. Start teaching your child that everyone goes to the potty throughout the day. Instead of keeping them on a strict time schedule and reminding them every 30 or so minutes, remind them to go potty prior to transitions. For instance, after they wake up on Day 2, invite them to go potty. After they finish a new activity or ask to go outside, prompt them to go potty first. Of course, if 45 to 60 minutes have passed since your child's last potty attempt, prompt them to use the potty. This is when you want to start phasing out time-based reminders and rely more on your child's body cues and normal daily transitions in determining when to prompt your child to go to the potty.

Step 4: Leave Your Home Commando Style

If you're feeling daring (or going crazy from being inside all day on Day 1) and you think both you and your child are ready, take your child on a brief outing. You'll know you're ready for an outing if on Day 1 your child had several successful eliminations and you both are beginning to develop a potty routine. Don't go too far, though! Keep your first outing short (around 15 to 30 minutes); go to a nearby park or run a quick errand. Have your child go commando and wear loose-fitting pants. You can say something like, "Be sure to keep your pants dry. Let me know if you get the potty feeling and need to go potty. I am bringing the travel potty for you to use while we're out." Pick an outing that does not have a time constraint (like an appointment at 10:00 a.m.) so your child uses the potty right before leaving home without rushing. Bring an extra change of clothes in case of accidents. A car seat/stroller cover also comes in handy for accidents while on the go. If your child remains dry throughout the entire outing, give them lots of praise (a treat is optional) and prompt them to go potty when you return home.

Day 3: Step-by-Step

In terms of technique, Day 3 will not be much different. The biggest change in Day 3 is to introduce underwear.

Step 1: Keep the Liquids and Salty Snacks Coming

Continue to give your child ample liquids, watery fruits, and salty snacks to give them plenty of opportunities to practice going to the potty.

IDEAS FOR TRIPS THAT TAKE
5 TO 10 MINUTES:

▶ Go outside and explore. Look for flowers, bugs, and rocks.

▶ Watch for clouds or planes passing by.

▶ Take a trip to the mailbox.

▶ Walk to the end of the block and back.

▶ Take the dog for a quick walk. This is great opportunity for potty talk.

IDEAS FOR TRIPS THAT TAKE
15 TO 30 MINUTES:

▶ Water play in the backyard.

▶ Walk a couple of blocks.

▶ Visit a nearby park.

▶ Run a quick errand.

▶ Clean out the car.

▶ Water plants or the grass.

Step 2: Introduce Underwear

If all is going (fairly) well and your child has had several successful eliminations on the potty, it's time to introduce underwear. Throughout the day, praise your child for keeping their underwear (or favorite character) dry and comfortable. This will help them make the connection between holding in their bowel or bladder movements with staying dry and feeling good. This is also a great way to subtly remind them to go to the potty as needed in a nonthreatening way. Keep it fun and light, and say something like, "It's potty time! Let's keep (favorite character) nice and dry." Keep in mind, however, that underwear can mimic the warm, snug feeling of diapers. If you notice your child having more accidents once you put on underwear, try going back to commando for a few more days (or weeks) until they have several successful eliminations on the potty.

Step 3: Leave Home

Plan another outing for Day 3. You can make it slightly longer this time (45 to 60 minutes), but don't go too far from home for too long. Just as on Day 2, have your child go to the potty beforehand (but don't rush them). Remind them of the travel potty and the importance of keeping their favorite character dry (if they're wearing underwear), and bring a change of underwear and pants just in case. If they remain dry throughout the entire outing, give them lots of praise and then prompt them to go potty when you return home.

Day 4 and Beyond

The days to come are more of the same. Keep the potty routine consistent. Continue to load up on liquids, watery fruits, and salty snacks until your child is consistently having successful eliminations on the potty. Gradually move toward less prompting, and praise your child for keeping their underwear dry and for self-initiating potty time. Follow your child's lead when trying to decide whether to move up a step. For instance, if they are continuing to have accidents throughout the day, it might not be time for a public outing or the introduction of underwear. Just as you were mindful of your child's developmental signs of readiness prior to beginning potty training, you need to be respectful of their ability to handle increased challenges. Move at their pace and adjust according to the feedback you get from them.

THINGS TO KEEP IN MIND FOR DAY 4 AND BEYOND:

▶ Stick with your potty routine.

▶ Continue to load up on liquids and salty snacks to continue practicing.

▶ Gradually move toward less and less prompting to promote your child's independence.

▶ Cut back on rewards once your child has several successes. A sticker chart (if you're using one) is usually the first thing to go. Also, once your child has mastered peeing on the potty, you can begin saving rewards for successful poop trips and/or going a whole day without accidents.

▶ Expect accidents.

The average time it takes to become fully potty trained is anywhere from a few days to several months or longer. There's no hard and fast rule on how long it should take your child to become fully potty trained. Remember, this is not a race and every child will complete this milestone in their own time.

Let's Talk About Poop

Don't be alarmed if your child does not poop in the potty during the first few days of training. Children simply don't get as many chances to practice pooping in the potty as they do urinating. Children also commonly wait until naptime or bedtime to poop or withhold their bowel movements altogether during this time.

The common causes of poop resistance are fear, desire for control, and/or constipation. Oftentimes, children view poop as an extension of themselves and are frightened to feel it and see it in the potty. It can also be scary for small children to hear the new sounds (like the splash of the water after an elimination) and feel the sensations that are involved in the process. To help with this, educate your child on the natural bodily functions of eating and drinking and then eliminating. Read them a baby anatomy book so that they can see how it all works. Also, continue to role-play their doll (or action figure or stuffed animal) going poop in the potty. Use a raisin to demonstrate how the toy pooped in the potty and have a celebration. If you feel comfortable, you can also help normalize this process by showing them your poop and saying bye-bye to it as you flush. Use intentional phrases like "slide out" and "let it out/let it go" to reinforce the idea that eliminating is an easy and natural thing to do.

Oftentimes, your child's resistance to poop stems from their need to take back control. And as frustrating as this may be, you can't force your child to poop in the potty. Avoid forcing your child to sit on the potty when they don't want to, because it can create more fear and resistance. Your child will poop in the potty when they feel comfortable enough to do so. When they poop in their naptime/nighttime pull-up (see Chapter 5), try not to get frustrated. Instead, involve your child in the process of putting the poop into the toilet and having them say bye-bye to it. Nonchalantly remind them: "Poop goes in the potty."

The best thing you can do is keep track of your child's poop schedule and encourage them to sit on the potty for around 10 minutes during the times they usually poop. Generally speaking, bowel movements occur 20 to 30 minutes after a meal; simply encourage them to sit on the potty then. Pooping in the potty is a matter of concentration too. Your child needs to be able to sit on the toilet long enough to have a bowel movement. Encourage them to sit for as long as it takes. You can give them an iPad, bubbles to blow, or something else for entertainment to help them stay seated. Keep in mind that pooping is a primal function that oftentimes requires privacy. A diaper offers that sense of privacy your child needs, so if your child appears resistant or anxious to poop in the potty, step away and allow them some privacy.

Also, make sure that your child is not constipated. Common signs of constipation include big, hard, and painful bowel movements, straining during bowel movements, and communicating fear related to using the potty due to pain. You can help alleviate constipation by increasing fluids and fiber in their diet. (See Chapter 9 for more information on constipation.)

Accidents

As messy as they are, accidents are inevitable and a natural part of the potty training process. They are actually the best way your child will learn how to go on the potty, because it provides them with the natural consequence of being wet and uncomfortable. When accidents happen (because they will), calmly tell yourself, "My child is one step closer to learning how to go on the potty." Most accidents happen because your child was busy playing or because they simply forgot. Although accidents can be frustrating, resist the urge to criticize or punish your child for them. This is counterproductive and increases the likelihood of future accidents due to stress.

Ideally, you will catch the accident in progress (you see your child urinating or defecating on the floor) because real-

To Sit or to Stand?

While boys are not necessarily harder to potty train, they tend to be ready to potty train slightly later than girls (usually a difference of months, not years) and can take a bit longer to master the new skill. It generally takes girls who are ready about 3 to 6 months to become fully potty trained, with boys tending to take a few months longer.

During the early stages of potty training, have your boy pee while sitting on the potty. Why? To keep things simple by teaching him to sit for both urination and bowel movements. If he stands, there will also be extra cleanup involved as he works on his aim. When teaching your boy to sit on the potty seat, direct him to spread his legs and push his penis straight down before he sits to avoid scraping it on the splash guard. Once your child masters sitting on the potty, you can begin to teach him how to pee standing if you're using a potty chair. However, there's no rush with this. He can pee sitting for as long as he likes. If you're using a toilet insert, you will need to make sure he is tall enough to successfully pee while standing. Use potty training targets (like Cheerios) or food coloring to teach aim and provide a little fun and motivation. It might also be helpful to involve a male family member (like dad, uncle, or grandpa) to show him how it's done.

As for girls, they will of course sit on the toilet for both peeing and pooping. Remember that you'll need to teach a girl to wipe from front to back to avoid getting feces into their urinary tract, which can lead to irritation and infection.

time experience is the best teacher. This is how remaining attentive to your child in the early days will pay off in the end. If you catch the accident in progress, quickly but calmly pick your child up and bring them to the potty. Once you arrive, say something like, "Pee and poop go in the potty." Praise them (and reward them if you're going this route) if they're able to get any amount of urine or feces in the potty. This is still an accomplishment to be celebrated.

After the potty routine is completed (wiping, flushing, pulling up pants, and washing and drying hands), involve your child in the cleanup process. If they defecate, have them help you bring the poop to the toilet and flush. Say calmly, "Pee and poop go in the potty. Where does it go? That's right, in the potty. Good job!" If you don't catch the accident in the moment, don't fret; you can still clean up with your child and remind them where pee and poop go. If your child told you about their accident, praise them for letting you know.

Don't say, "It's okay," because although you want to communicate to your child that you understand and are not upset with them for having an accident, you don't want to send the message that it's okay to have an accident. Instead, gently remind them that pee and poop go in the potty and that they can try again later. Then clean up and move on as quickly as possible.

You might also go back to prompting every 30 to 60 minutes and/or setting a timer if you notice that accidents are becoming more frequent. Continue reading potty books and role-play with a doll if that has been helpful in the past. Also, consider whether your child may be constipated. Accidents are more common if constipation is present (see Chapter 9).

Hygiene Practices

It's important to teach your child good hygiene practices at the start of the journey. Model hand washing after you use the toilet, explaining that it gets rid of germs that can make them sick. Point out any dirt on their hands and under their nails, then point out how clean their hands look once they're done with hand washing. Keep this conversation simple and matter-of-fact. Keep fun pump soaps handy in the bathroom and sing songs like "The Wheels on the Bus" or "Row, Row, Row Your Boat" while washing to encourage your child to wash long enough (around 20 seconds). Have them wash both sides of their hands and in between their fingers. After hand washing, help them dry their hands.

Wiping is usually the last skill to be mastered. Teach this skill early in the process so your child knows wiping is an important step (just like flushing and hand washing). Show your child how much toilet paper to use. A good rule of thumb is to have them measure from their fingers to their elbow. Also, tell them to wipe from front to back (especially girls). After urination, teach them to pat clean and dry.

The wiping process will take much more effort and instruction on your part when it comes to poop. At first you will do the dirty work and then have your child participate in the second go-around. You will want them to look at the toilet paper (or flushable wipe) after they wipe, and tell them to wipe until they no longer see a brown stain. Some children learn best by squatting down and touching their toes so that their cheeks easily spread. You may need to tell your child to put the dirty toilet paper in the toilet after each wipe to avoid smearing the poop, and flush.

Keep in mind that your child might not have the motor skills necessary to achieve the correct wiping motion, especially for cleaning up poop. Set realistic expectations, and always model how to wipe their bottoms first. After all, wiping is less intuitive than using the potty, so set realistic expectations, give clear instructions, and give them lots of opportunities to practice. Most preschool teachers do not get involved in the wiping process, so this is an important skill for your child to know before going into that setting.

And, of course, you also want to speak to your child about the importance of flushing. Some kids might be a little scared of the flushing sound at first, but most become comfortable with it after a few times.

Looking Back and Moving Forward

Let's recap the major points of this chapter:

▶ This potty training program is designed to be as simple and straightforward as possible while also being flexible. There is no one-size-fits-all approach, so adjust the program as necessary.

▶ Be positive, clear, and consistent in your approach, stay attentive, and try to enjoy the process as much as possible.

▶ The program is broken down into a 3-day step-by-step process, with Day 4 and beyond following the same steps.

▶ On **Day 1,** have your child go naked from the waist down. Load them up on liquids and watch them like a hawk. Prompt your child to go to the potty every 20 to 30 minutes, and then gradually lengthen the time between prompts. Praise your child for their successes and remain calm during the inevitable accidents.

▶ On **Day 2,** continue all practices from Day 1 and add a short public outing (no longer than 30 minutes) if you and your child are ready for the challenge. Bring the travel potty and a change of clothes, and praise your child if they are able to keep their pants dry.

▶ **Day 3** is more of the same, but adding a slightly longer public outing (45 to 60 minutes) and underwear if you two are ready. Over time, you will want to create and maintain a potty routine that is built around natural transitions.

- ▶ Don't be alarmed if your child does not poop in the toilet during the first few days of potty training. Encourage them to sit on the potty 20 to 30 minutes after meals, and give them lots of entertainment to help them sit long enough to have a bowel movement. Offer privacy if your child appears anxious or resistant.

- ▶ There are slight differences when it comes to potty training boys and girls centered around readiness, length of time it takes to potty train, and hygiene practices.

- ▶ Accidents are an inevitable part of the process. Remind them that pee and poop go in the potty and not on the floor, involve them in the cleanup process, and then move on.

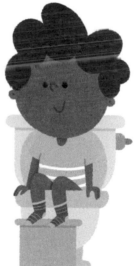

- ▶ Involve your child in hygiene practices early on.

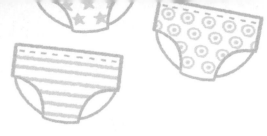

CHAPTER 5

Naps and Nighttime Training

SO, YOUR CHILD IS well on their way to accident-free daytime potty training—but what's happening at naps and at night? You may need to adopt new strategies for times of sleep.

Naps

While daytime potty training readiness depends on a host of developmental factors, including physiological, psychological, motor, and cognitive development, naptime training readiness is solely dependent on physiological development. Basically, your child's ability to stay dry during naps and bedtime is based on their bladder development. While your child may be advanced cognitively and emotionally, their bladder might not be able to physically handle the task of holding urine and/or sending a wake-up message to the brain. Also, some children are not awakened by the elimination sensation because they sleep so deeply or are not as sensitive to the sensation of being wet. (In other words, naptime and bedtime accidents are almost always involuntary.) Sleep and bladder sensations mature over time, so wait until your child has fully mastered daytime potty training and is waking up several times in a row with a dry diaper before you begin naptime potty training. Remember, naptime training usually comes well after daytime success.

In the meantime, have your child sit on the potty before napping. Put your child in a pull-up, but make sure it looks completely different from their diapers. Tell them they have now graduated to "naptime underpants." If they have a character on them, use the character's name to describe what they are ("princess underpants," for example). Tell them to try to keep their "naptime underpants" dry. When they wake up, check the pull-up and praise your child if they were able to keep them dry. Remember, this will come with time. Putting too much emphasis on the outcome can overwhelm your child and make them feel bad about themselves. It is imperative that you remove their pull-up *immediately* after naptime to avoid any confusion.

Once your child has had several dry pull-ups after naps (at least three in a row), then you can begin naptime potty training. Always have your child go potty just prior to naps. Put their underwear on and then their pull-up so that they can feel when they've had an accident. Once they're able to accomplish another stretch of dryness with their underwear and pull-up, then it's safe to ditch the pull-up. Place a plastic cover over their mattress and put them in underwear for naptime. Tell them to try to keep their character underwear dry and reward them for dryness after naps.

If your child has several accidents at naptime, return to underwear and pull-ups. This may be a sign your child is not fully physiological ready yet, and that's okay. Take a break and try again later.

Nighttime

Dr. T. Berry Brazelton, pediatrician and founder of the child-oriented approach to potty training, said it best: "In the toilet training arena, staying dry at night is a child's crowning achievement." Nighttime success will come much later than daytime and naptime achievement. As noted earlier, your child's ability to stay dry throughout the night is largely dependent on their physiological development.

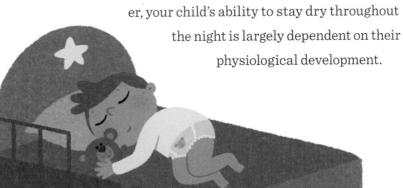

What About Naps in the Car?

Car rides and traveling while potty training can feel daunting, especially if your child tends to nap during trips. Try to avoid accidents in the car by prompting your child to go potty right before leaving home, limiting drinks before and during the car ride, and making car rides brief. You can also try to prevent naps by keeping your child engaged by creating a fun atmosphere through singing, playing upbeat music, having conversations about where you're going, and playing simple games, such as "I Spy," to keep your child engaged.

Sometimes, though, naps are unavoidable, so use a car seat protector in case of accidents. And for longer car rides, consider placing your child in a pull-up and then taking it off immediately upon arrival. (See more about traveling while potty training in Chapter 8.)

Generally speaking, children become nighttime potty trained when they either have the ability to wake up during the night to relieve themselves or they have a big enough bladder to hold urine until the morning. A good indicator that your child is ready to begin nighttime training is if they are nearly fully daytime potty trained (with infrequent accidents), successful at keeping dry during naps, and are waking up in a dry pull-up in the morning for several mornings at a time.

Children tend to achieve nighttime success anywhere from 6 months to 1 year (or longer) after they become day-time trained. Most children can stay dry throughout the night by age 5. (Bedtime accidents—bedwetting—occur in 20 percent of 5-year-old children and 10 to 15 percent of 6-year-old children. Bedwetting tends to be more common among boys, with 7 out of 10 bedwetters being male.) Again, nighttime accidents are commonly a result of physiological reasons, including small bladder size, muscle relaxation during sleep, and an inability to recognize the need to elimi-nate while sleeping.

When to Start Nighttime Training

A good rule of thumb is to wait at least 6 months after your child is fully daytime potty trained (including naptime) before working on nighttime training. You will also want to be on the lookout for several dry pull-ups in the morning to signal that your child is ready.

Here are other factors that show your child is ready for nighttime training:

▶ Your child asks to sleep without a pull-up.
▶ Your child sleeps in a toddler bed and has easy access to the toilet throughout the night.
▶ Your child has the motor skills necessary to get out of bed, as well as push down and pull up their pants independently.
▶ Your child understands the feeling of needing to go and regularly initiates potty trips on their own.

What should you do while you wait for signs of physiological readiness?

▶ Stick to your daytime potty routine. Nighttime training stems from daytime practices, so stay consistent in your potty routine.
▶ Be intentional about liquids. Give your child plenty of liquids during the daytime and taper down drinks after dinner. In particular, limit juice and other sugary drinks 2 hours before bedtime because they tend to bring more water into the bladder.

- ▶ Add potty trips to the bedtime routine. Have your child go potty during the bedtime routine (around 30 minutes prior to bedtime, such as after bath time) and then again immediately right before bedtime.
- ▶ Use nighttime pull-ups while you wait for your child to show signs of readiness. Just as with naps, call them "nighttime underpants" and remove them immediately after they wake up. Some children will remain dry throughout the night only to urinate right after they wake up. To prevent this, wake your child up 10 to 15 minutes before they usually rise, remove the pull-up, and have them go potty.

Once Your Child Shows Signs of Physiological Readiness

When your child demonstrates they are ready by waking up dry several mornings in a row, put them in underwear and then nighttime pull-ups (just as you did for naptime). When they continue to stay dry during nighttime, ditch the pull-ups and opt for underwear only.

If your child wakes up dry, praise them but hold off on the rewards. Oftentimes, naptime and nighttime success is achieved without conscious control, and you don't want to reward what your child can't control. Show your happiness with a simple "Good job!" and move on.

Be Prepared for Accidents

Be prepared for accidents by placing a waterproof cover on your child's mattress and double layer the sheets. Place a waterproof cover over the mattress, then a sheet, then another plastic cover, and one more sheet on top. That way, if your child has an accident, you can simply strip off the top two layers and the bed is ready for your child again. You can use baking soda or eucalyptus oil to remove the urine odor from sheets and clothing.

Be patient and nonchalant when accidents happen. Remember, it can take up to a year for your child to stay dry all night, every night. However, if your child has consistent accidents for a couple of weeks straight, this may be a sign they are not physiologically ready. Return to pull-ups and try again at a later time.

An Alternative Method for Nighttime Training

Some parents prefer waking their child up either 60 to 90 minutes after they have fallen asleep, right before the parent goes to bed, or during the middle of the night for a "dream pee." While this strategy probably does not speed up the child's physiological development and may actually hinder the correct brain signals from developing, it does lead to fewer accidents throughout the night. This option is recommended only if your child's sleep is not significantly impacted and they are able to easily go back to sleep. Remember, just as with daytime training strategies, you can always change your mind and switch up your approach if you notice it's not working for either you or your child.

When Is Bedwetting a Problem?

Generally speaking, pediatricians say bedwetting occurs when a child is at least 5 years old and having nighttime accidents more than once a week for at least a 3-month span. You'll want to consult your doctor if your child is 7 years or older and wetting the bed more than two to three times per week. Bedwetting prior to age 7 is not generally thought of as a cause for concern, as your child is likely still developing nighttime bladder control. With time, most children will outgrow bedwetting on their own.

CONSULT YOUR CHILD'S PEDIATRICIAN IF:

▶ Your child is 7 years old or older and bedwetting a couple of times per week for months at a time.

▶ Your child shows signs of regression: bedwetting after a few months of staying dry through the night.

▶ Your child complains of pain while urinating, exhibits unusual thirst, has pink or red urine or hard stools, or is snoring (since sleep apnea can interfere with sleep and consequently with nighttime potty training).

Keep in mind that bedwetting tends to run in families and can be due to a sleep disorder or disruptions related to medical issues such as sleep apnea, a urinary tract infection, problems with the ureters, tonsillar or adenoidal hypertrophy, or other issues. Stress can also be a factor in bedwetting. Your child's pediatrician will be able to determine whether your child's bedwetting is due to a medical issue. Interventions such as a bedwetting alarm system, treating constipation (if applicable), and/or medication may be beneficial for your child. Consult with your child's pediatrician if the strategies outlined in this chapter have not worked and you're interested in other options. Prior to your appointment, keep track of your child's eating and drinking patterns, how many bedwetting accidents they've had in the past several weeks, and how often they urinate.

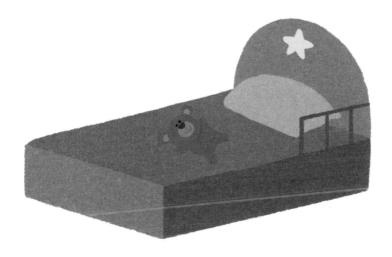

Looking Back and Moving Forward

Let's recap the major points of this chapter:

▶ Your child's readiness for naptime and bedtime potty training will be largely dependent on their physiological development. Your child should be fully daytime potty trained (including naps) and waking up dry consistently for several mornings before nighttime training.

▶ Put your child in pull-ups and remove them immediately after your child wakes up and have them sit on the potty.

▶ When it comes to naptime training, start by placing them in underwear and then a pull-up. If they continue to consistently wake up dry, ditch the pull-ups. Place double layers of waterproof covers and sheets on their mattress for added protection.

▶ Once your child has mastered naptime training for several weeks, it may be time for bedtime training. Develop a bedtime routine that includes limiting drinks after dinner, going to the potty 30 minutes prior to bedtime, and then going again right before bedtime. Consider waking up your child 10 to 15 minutes prior to their usual wake-up time to prevent accidents.

▶ It can take up to a year for your child to be able to stay dry all night, every night. Most children are fully nighttime trained by 5 years old. Try to stay patient when accidents happen, trusting your child will develop this skill when they are developmentally ready.

CHAPTER 6

What about My Child?

SO, YOU'VE GOT THE BASICS under control, but your child isn't completely on board yet. Personality traits, developmental delays, and special situations can affect potty training. With these unique situations comes the risk of falling into power struggles. Here's what to do to maintain the parent–child relationship and continue along the potty training path.

Strong-Willed Children

Strong-willed, stubborn, and spirited children can be a challenge to potty train; at the same time, they are likely to be highly self-motivated and inner-directed, which can work to your advantage. They are courageous and independent, wanting to learn things in their own way and in their own time. Because of this, they tend to test limits in an attempt to learn things their own way. They may also have big, passionate feelings. Remember, it takes two to have a power struggle. You can disengage by validating their emotions while holding firm limits. You can say something like, "I see. You don't want to wash your hands right now. I get it." You want to truly connect with your child and let them know you understand and sympathize with their frustration before trying to get them to cooperate with you.

After validating their emotions, move on to strategies for compliance. Redirect their behavior by saying something like, "Yes, I see you need my help washing your hands," and then gently yet firmly hold their hands under the water. Try to keep this process upbeat by singing a fun song or describing what you're doing. For instance, you can say something like, "Wash, wash those germs away. Bye-bye germs!" Over time, your

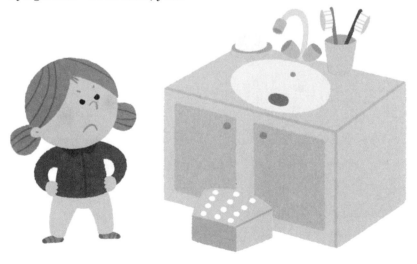

child should resist less if you keep this process positive. Praise your child when you're done by saying something like, "Yeah, I get it. You don't like washing your hands. Thanks for letting me help you." And then move on as quickly as possible. You don't want to draw attention to the undesired behavior.

There are a few other strategies you can use to give your strong-willed child some control without compromising your goal of complying with the potty routine.

Give Two Choices

Offering two choices is one of your best strategies for potty training your strong-willed child (or any child for that matter). This approach lets you both have some control. For instance, you can give your child the choice of which underwear to put on, where to place the potty in your home, whether to go to the potty in 2 minutes or 5 minutes, what kind of juice to drink, whether or not they would like your help in dressing and undressing, and even where to go during your public outing.

In every situation, give your child only two choices (so you don't overwhelm them) and make sure both of those choices are equally fine with you. It's frustrating and confusing to be told to make a choice only to hear you picked the wrong one. So, for example, if you want your child to choose where to go on your short outing, you can say something like, "We are going to leave home soon. Would you like to go to the library or the park?" In other circumstances, you can say, "You have two choices: You can undress yourself or I can help you" or "It's time to put on your underwear. Would you like the Superman ones or the Batman ones?" or "It's time to sit on the potty. Would you like to read a book or play with this toy while you go?" It's incredibly rewarding for children to be empowered by the gift of choices.

Use When/Then Statements

Using *when/then* statements is another great way to get your child on board and gain greater cooperation. Use *when/then* statements when you need your child to do something first before moving on to another activity or receiving a reward. For instance, you would say something like, "It's almost time to leave for the park. *When* you go potty, *then* it will be time to go." Or if your child went on the potty and you need their cooperation in flushing and hand washing before moving on to the next activity, you could say something like, "It's bath time! *When* you flush and wash your hands, *then* you can take a bath."

When using *when/then* statements, you must not move on to the next activity before your child has done what you told them to do. This is key to instilling trust and letting your child know you mean what you say. So, for instance, you would not leave home until they have at least sat on the potty and made an effort to go.

Overall, with strong-willed children, you want to always be clear when it comes to your expectations and use *when/then* statements to convey them clearly and calmly.

Focus on Your Connection

If your relationship with your child has taken a beating from potty training, focus on connection. You are more likely to gain your child's cooperation when you have a strong, warm relationship with them. Get down on your child's level every day and simply play with them. This will go a long way toward enhancing your relationship—and toward setting the stage for successful potty training.

Take a Step Back

If your child is resistant to even sitting on the potty, you'll need to take a step back. You can't expect them to use the potty until they are comfortable with sitting on it long enough to go. Start with small steps and use small rewards (like one gummy bear or fruit snack) when they sit on the potty. Once they've shown they are comfortable, reward them for using the potty. Try to avoid getting upset with your child for resisting the potty and use the *when/then* approach to gain their cooperation. For instance, say, "When you sit on the potty, then you get to choose a toy from the basket." Praise their small successes and trust in the process as much as possible.

If you have a strong-willed child on your hands, potty

training will take an extra strong dose of patience. Resist the urge to give up and go back to diapers. If you've deemed your child developmentally ready for potty training, then stick with it. Your strong-willed child will get it eventually.

Anxious Children

Potty training an anxious child can be frustrating for all parties involved. The process may be stalled until you're able to understand the root of your child's anxiety and help them work through it. In the meantime, hold off on giving rewards if your child is not able to earn them. Nothing is more frustrating and shame-inducing than not being able to earn a reward because relentless fear gets in the way.

Your child may fear some aspect of the toilet itself, such as the flushing noise. If your child has experienced pain while urinating or during a bowel movement from being constipated, they may develop potty-related anxiety. It takes only one painful pooping episode for your child to avoid the potty altogether. (If you suspect your child is constipated, see Chapter 9 for more information.)

If you think your child's anxiety is rooted in some aspect of the toilet, take a step back and return to the basics discussed in Chapter 2. In particular, you'll want to return to potty training books to normalize the experience, and baby anatomy books if you suspect your child has fears related to eliminating. And don't forget that play is a powerful tool you can use to help your child explore, communicate, and process their anxious feelings. Encourage your child to play with a doll around the potty and see if you can explore their potty-related anxieties.

If your child is adamant about not using the potty, you may want to try a process known as *gradual exposure*. To help alleviate your child's anxiety, gradually expose them to anxiety-provoking situations and help them calm down. This process is done in small steps and at your child's pace. You will want to start with the least anxiety-provoking situations and then gradually work your way up. For instance, start by reading and watching videos about going to the potty. Then begin playing with a doll or action figure around their toy toilet. Praise the doll for being brave and going to the potty. Act out scenes where the doll is anxious and talk about how they calmed down (by taking deep breaths, asking for help, counting to 10, taking a break) and continued to go potty despite their fears.

Next, bring the doll or action figure into the bathroom or near your child's potty chair. While playing, suggest your child sit on the potty but don't force it. Make this fun and playful, and always follow your child's lead. For instance, you could say, "Wow! The doll was so brave. She used the potty even though she was scared." Wait a while and then say, "I wonder if you could try to sit on the potty just like the doll did." If your child complies, praise them and emphasize how brave and courageous they are and how safe and comfortable the potty chair is. If they resist, don't worry. This process could take several days before you see any progress. The idea is to continue exposing your child to the stressor and helping them work through their anxiety either in indirect (play) or direct (sit on the potty chair) ways.

With anxious children, consider small tweaks like changing to a potty chair if the flushing noise is bothersome. You may also want to transfer them to a potty chair if they are afraid of the adult toilet. Try to determine the root of their anxiety so that you can intervene accordingly. If your child continues exhibiting anxiety related to going potty after trying the above-mentioned strategies, consider consulting with a counselor or mental health professional for more personalized guidance.

Late Bloomers

There's such a wide age range for hitting developmental milestones, and it's completely normal for children to vary in terms of abilities, motivation, and pace. Potty training is no exception. Some children master it slower than others, and that's okay. Your child will learn new skills at their own pace and in their own way. If you've deemed them developmentally ready and checked with their pediatrician and ruled out any medical causes (like constipation) for potty training delays, then it's time to trust in the process.

If your child is a late bloomer, you may be dismayed when you compare their potty training journey to that of other children you know. But here's the thing many first-time parents (in fact, all parents) might need to remember: Raising kids is not a competitive sport, and just because your child learns developmental milestones later than other children does not mean you've failed. It also doesn't mean your child has failed. Children can sense when you're trying to rush them to do something. Pressuring your child will cause stress for both of you. Children late to potty training need extra doses of encouragement and confidence. Here's what else you can do for your late bloomer.

Prepare and Prepare Some More

In addition to embracing your late bloomer and trusting they will learn in their own time, you can give them extra preparation before you actually try to get them to use the potty. Simply reading books on potty training and practicing with their doll or action figure can go a long way in demystifying the process, preparing, and motivating your child for potty training. Sing potty training songs. Provide "learning moments" throughout the day by bringing them into the bathroom with you and providing running commentary about what you're doing.

Try a New Approach

If potty training has been delayed because your child is not interested in sitting on the potty, it's time to try a new approach. Simply remind your child that the character on their underwear doesn't like to get poop and pee on them, so it's their job to get rid of both in the potty—and then stop talking about it. Stop reminding them. Reminders can feel like pressure to a resistant child. Don't accompany them to the bathroom unless they request your presence. Approach accidents neutrally and enlist their help cleaning up the mess in a matter-of-fact way. Get them involved in changing out of their soiled clothes and picking out new underwear and pants. However, avoid treating the cleanup process like a punishment for their accident. Instead, view it as a natural consequence for making a mess. Reward your child every time they use the toilet, and give lots of praise and physical affection (hugs, kisses, high fives, pats on the back). Let them know just how proud you are of them becoming a big kid.

Ask for Help

Parents of late bloomers often grow frustrated and out of patience. Potty training may have become a much longer journey than you were prepared for, and it's easy to feel like you're failing as a parent. It may be time to give yourself a potty training break and enlist the support of other caregivers to help. Taking a break can give you a fresh new perspective and help you muster up more patience and positivity. Your child may also benefit from learning from someone new.

Whose Delay?

It's time to be honest with yourself. Is your child truly a late bloomer, or are you avoiding the process? If you think your child's potty training delays have more to do with your own avoidance, you'll need to regroup and take small steps toward preparing yourself for the journey ahead. You're already doing great by reading this book!

> **Be honest with yourself about your fears of potty training.**

Be honest with yourself about your fears of potty training, and challenge your negative beliefs as much as you can. For instance, are you telling yourself that potty training is going to be hard and messy? Do you lack faith in your child's ability to learn the skill? Or do you not have enough faith in yourself? Next, ask yourself, "Are these beliefs accurate?" and "Are these helpful thoughts to have? Do they move me closer to my goal of getting my child potty trained?"

Finally, ask yourself, "What are some more helpful thoughts I can have about potty training that will move me and my child forward?" Spend time reflecting on your current state of mind, and take steps toward adjusting it to be more realistic and positive. A positive mindset will go a

Help Wanted!

Many first-time parents think they must do everything on their own, so they're reluctant to ask for help when they really need it. But the simple truth is, sometimes it's hard for kids to take direction from their primary caregivers. In fact, some children might be more likely to listen to how awesome the potty is from other family members, such as grandma or grandpa, their favorite aunt or uncle, or an older (and maybe cooler) cousin.

And when you're stuck inside for those first few days, don't be shy about calling in reinforcements to offer assistance so you can run out for a coffee or take a quick walk around the block for some much-needed "me time."

long way in minimizing your avoidance, committing to the journey, and being successful.

Children with Special Needs

Potty training can be difficult under any circumstances, but potty training a child with special needs can feel like a daunting task that won't ever get done. It's important to keep in mind that children with special needs commonly begin potty training later than other children. It can also take them up to age 5 or later to complete the process. In addition, children with severe physical disabilities may require assistance with removing clothing and accessing the bathroom indefinitely.

You will want to start the potty training process by first determining whether your child is developmentally ready (See Chapter 1 for more information.) Always keep in mind that children, especially those with special needs, move at their own pace. Forcing them to do things they are not ready for is not only a waste of time but is also incredibly frustrating for everyone involved. On the other hand, while you never want to push your child to do things they are incapable of, persevering during challenges can have an enormous impact on your child's self-esteem. Only you can know what's right for your child.

Prior to beginning, there are a few things to do if your child has special needs. First, enlist help from your partner, relatives, or friends to help boost morale and ensure you're not doing this alone. You'll also want to consult with your child's pediatrician and other providers who may be involved in your child's care. They will be able to provide a physical assessment, offer specific recommendations related to your child's unique needs, and give you information about special equipment you may need before you get started.

Speech Delays

One of the biggest difficulties in potty training children with speech delays is communicating the need to go. If you've determined that your child is developmentally ready but they have difficulties with speech, you'll need to establish a simple form of communication you both understand. Pick one sign or gesture for needing to eliminate, and use this every time your child goes on the potty. Some examples include signals for *pee, poop, potty,* or *need to go.* This could mean teaching them sign language, such as how to sign *potty.* Be flexible, and simplify the signs to accommodate your child's little hands and fingers. Also, if your child adapts a sign to fit their needs, let them. Check in with your child's speech pathologist for ideas of words and gestures to use.

Another strategy is to use tangible symbols or have them point to symbols on a piece of paper. For instance, you can keep a tangible symbol that represents the bathroom (like a piece of tile if your bathroom has tiles) handy for your child to refer to. You can also hang up a picture of a toilet for your child to point to when they need to go potty.

Children with Visual Impairment

If your child is visually impaired, you should wait to start until their language skills are well-developed. Take them to their potty and give them plenty of opportunities to explore the bathroom (or areas where their potty chairs are located). Invite them to the bathroom with you, and provide lots of commentary on what you're doing and why. Guide their hands to all the toileting components, like the toilet paper dispenser, flush handle, and sink. Keep the potty in the same location, and keep the path to it clear of obstacles. You may also want to purchase a potty that plays music when urine touches the bowl to help add hearing fun to the process.

Children with Hearing Impairment

If your child has a hearing impairment, you will want to teach them essential signs, such as *wet*, *dry*, and *need to go* before beginning the potty training process. You can start by using these signs every time you go to the restroom and during diaper changes. Be consistent until they can successfully demonstrate the signs on their own. Once your child has the essential signs down, begin teaching them other important signs, including pushing down and pulling up pants, wiping, flushing, and hand washing. Throughout this process, be aware that their body language also signals that they need to eliminate. Praise them for their efforts in communicating with you and reinforce potty signs as often as you can. For example, you can use the sign for *need to go* while your child

> **Visual aids, including modeling the potty process for your child, reading books, and showing them pictures, are great ways to teach your child about potty training.**

is demonstrating the nonverbal cues to help them learn to associate these signs with their bodily sensations. Visual aids, including modeling the potty process for your child, reading books, and showing them pictures, are great ways to teach your child about potty training. Create a picture sequence—such as walk to bathroom, push down pants, sit down and wait, wipe, pull up pants, flush, and wash hands—to help them learn the potty process. Have these pictures in the bathroom for your child to regularly refer back to.

Intellectual and Developmental Delays

If your child has an intellectual and/or developmental delay, the potty training process will depend largely on your child's individual personality, any coexisting conditions, and their patterns of behavior. You will want to keep in mind your child's unique strengths, weaknesses, interests, and way of learning—and be mindful that you might have to move a bit slower with the overall process depending on your child's method of learning. For instance, some children with developmental disorders have difficulty imitating the behaviors of others, while some may learn best through simple imitation and nonverbal demonstrations.

Begin by rewarding successive steps, such as simply walking into the bathroom, sitting on the toilet with pants, then without pants, and finally eliminating. You can save teaching your child how to push down and pull up their underwear and pants for when they have successfully mastered the bathroom routine. If your child has limited verbal abilities, you'll need to handle accidents in a firm, matter-of-fact way and keep your instructions simple, such as, "Wet! Time to change!"

For children with developmental and intellectual delays, the process of potty training becomes easier once they are able to manage their clothing (though they may continue to need your help); can communicate, even if minimally; and can demonstrate awareness that they need to eliminate. Throughout the process, keep your language, including your explanations and prompts, as simple as possible. You may start by checking their diaper every 30 minutes or so and saying one word, such as *wet*. If their diaper is dry, smile and say, "Dry!" after you change them. When modeling the potty routine with your child, you can smile and tell them, "Dry!" Your child may make the connection between themselves and other children faster than with you, so expose them to videos and books related to potty training. Your child may also benefit from being able to practice the potty routine with a doll or action figure. Once your child is ready to use the potty, use the strategies in Chapter 4 and consult your pediatrician (and other involved providers) with any questions or concerns.

POTTY MOTIVATORS

Keep potty motivators in a basket in the bathroom to maintain your child's concentration and help them relax long enough to eliminate. Don't let your child play with them unless they're seated on the potty. These items are used to motivate, not to reward or provide entertainment outside of potty time. Potty motivators include the following:

- ▶ Your child's favorite music
- ▶ Album of family photos
- ▶ Sensory fidget toys
- ▶ Liquid motion bubbler timer
- ▶ Squeeze balls
- ▶ Musical toys
- ▶ Whistles
- ▶ Bubbles
- ▶ Picture books
- ▶ Plastic toys such as alphabet letters

Children with special needs often greatly benefit from a personalized potty story, because it gives them a clear understanding of what is expected of them as well as their reward for completing the desired action. Potty stories must be age-appropriate, relevant to your child, and straight to the point in order to be effective. Real-life pictures often work best; you can place the photographs in an accessible and portable album. Highlight the most important words so that you and your child can easily focus on the most important parts of the story. Read the potty story to your child throughout the day. If your child is in school, make a duplicate potty story so they can generalize their learning across different environments.

Another tip is to provide your child with a visual aid to remind them of the sequence of events when using the potty and of what happens after they go potty (the reward). For instance, place a picture of a potty with the word *First* at the top and then a picture of candy (or whatever reward you're using) next to it with the word *Then*. Keep this poster in the bathroom and other common areas of your home. Your child might also benefit from having a few pictures that illustrate the sequence of events when they use the potty. For example, you can have a picture of a child pushing pants down, sitting, going pee or poop, and then flushing. Make sure the poster only incorporates three to four pictures that are easy to follow and do not involve too many words. Point to the pictures and prompt your child for what comes next to help them stay involved in the process. You may also choose to laminate these pictures and bring them with you on outings as a helpful reminder.

Two Children (or More!) at a Time

Potty training two children (or more) involves many of the same steps you've learned so far. For instance, you'll want to ensure that each child is developmentally ready to begin potty training. Evaluate your children—individually—to determine the right timing. Remember, your children are separate people and may not be ready at the same time. For some children, potty training simultaneously is beneficial for the companionship and healthy competition, while for others it's too distracting and disruptive. Certainly, it's probably easiest to train all children at the same time, but you'll have to decide what to do based on each child's developmental readiness and their interpersonal dynamics.

If you end up potty training both children at the same time, try to enlist the support of another person (one for each child you're potty training). Having two sets of hands (or more) is the easiest way to train two (or more) children at once. Also, purchase lots and lots of underwear and one potty chair for each child (all identical and one for each child for each floor of your house). Don't let one child claim a potty as their own. If rewards are involved, determine what is reinforcing for each of your children. When one child gets a treat, tell the other(s) to at least sit on the potty if they also ask for one. This way, you're not creating resentment while you're sticking with the potty routine.

One thing to stay away from when tandem training: sticker charts. They will serve as a visual reminder that one child is performing "better" than the other(s). Some parents prefer to skip small treats and rewards altogether and stick with a silly, celebratory dance so all children can be involved. Find what works best for your children (and your sanity).

Be mindful of your children's individual needs, and remember you are potty training two (or more) different humans. Adjust your approach for each child, as their learning style and preferences may be very different. For example, some children love lots of praise, while others do not. Some children are open to their body functions, while others are more modest and prefer privacy. While some children appreciate reminders, others prefer to control the process and go in their own time.

> **Adjust your approach for each child, as their learning style and preferences may be very different.**

Don't use one child's success to motivate the other(s). This will only intensify feelings of jealousy and inadequacy, which can cause regression. Instead, look for success in all children and focus on the positives of all. If one child is progressing at a quicker rate than the other(s), keep going and focus more of your attention on getting that child potty trained first. Typically, the second or third child will catch up and become more interested once they see the other child(ren) having so much success.

Transitions and Training

Since potty training is a huge transition for the whole family, it's best not to begin the process during other major family changes such as a family vacation, divorce, death of a loved one, changes in work schedules, or shortly before or right after the birth of a new sibling. However, this is not always possible to avoid. When dealing with transitions and other special family situations while also potty training, avoid setting deadlines and be prepared for your child to regress. Potty training regression is common during times of stress and change. For this reason, it may be necessary to take a break from potty training if your child is regressing significantly. Wait until the situation has settled and your child is less stressed to resume potty training.

Potty training may need to be put on hold when one parent moves out of the home during a divorce. Though it's possible to potty train your child when they live in two homes, you'll need to first allow your child time to adjust to the changes. If your child appears to be having a hard time adjusting to the divorce, consider bringing up potty training later so you're not overwhelming them with too many new things at once.

When potty training during divorce, do your best to maintain communication with your former spouse and adhere to the same schedule at both households. It's best for your child if all parties agree on one strategy, since inconsistencies can lead to behavioral issues and confusion. If rewards are involved, keep them consistent. For instance, have two of the same sticker charts, and if you're using small treats, do so at both households. Buy two sets of potty training items, including underwear and pull-ups. If you started potty training and then stopped during the divorce, restart it the same way to make the adjustment easier. Make sure your child's experience at your home is positive and consistent. Children are remarkably resilient and will master potty training with time and extra patience, even if the two households are not perfectly aligned.

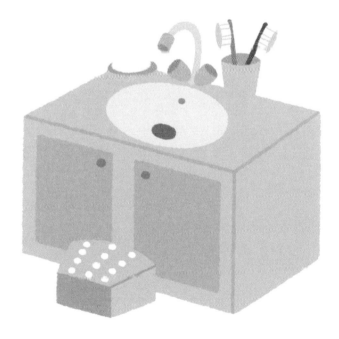

Looking Back and Moving Forward

Let's recap the major points of this chapter:

▶ Personality traits, developmental delays, and special situations can affect potty training.

▶ When potty training strong-willed children, eliminate power struggles by implementing lots of choices and *when/then* statements.

▶ If your child is anxious about this journey, you'll need to determine the root of their worry so that you can intervene appropriately. You can also use a process known as *gradual exposure* to slowly help your child through their fears.

▶ If you have a late bloomer, potty training may take longer than anticipated.

▶ Potty training children with special needs often takes longer than other children. Enlist the support of family and friends, and consult with your child's pediatrician and other treatment providers to help you determine when your child is ready to begin potty training.

▶ When potty training two children (or more!), determine their developmental readiness individually. When potty training at the same time, avoid comparisons, purchase one potty chair per floor for each child, and reward them based on what is reinforcing for each unique child.

- Ideally, potty training will not begin when stress levels are high. That means holding off during major family transitions such as moves, changes in work schedules, death of a loved one, and divorce.

- If you are potty training during divorce, try to maintain open communication with your former spouse and decide on one strategy to use. If not possible, be sure to provide consistency and positivity at your home.

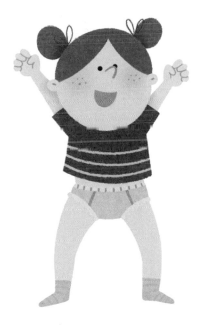

Beyond the Bathroom

Maybe potty training so far has been smooth sailing— or maybe it hasn't. And if it hasn't, there's no need to panic, but there may be call for additional advice. You might also need to know how to enlist potty training help for when you're not around. Check out the pages that follow for more tailored advice on what to do.

CHAPTER 7

Day Care and Other Caregiving Situations

IN AN IDEAL WORLD, you would be able to stay home when potty training your child. But that isn't reality for many parents, and let's be honest—it would be so much easier with support. So, let's look at how to enlist other caregivers to help potty train.

Day Care

Generally speaking, it's best to potty train your child in the absence of a big change such as a new day care. Try to wait until your child has settled into their new caregiving arrangement prior to starting this new journey. (If you can't wait, begin potty training at least 4 days before starting day care.) If you plan to begin potty training after your child starts their new day care, ask the day-care providers about their procedures and policies during your interview. Also, read their potty training policy and ask plenty of questions before you sign the day-care agreement. Some day-care providers require your child to be out of diapers and almost accident-free, while others will help you with the process. You'll want to be aware of their expectations prior to enrolling your child.

If your child's day care will be involved in potty training, ensure that you're on the same page and can maintain open communication throughout the process. Potty training a child in day care is a team effort. Ideally, parents and day-care providers will agree on an approach that works best for the child. After all, a consistent strategy can minimize your child's confusion and frustration. However, try to be flexible and know you can't change their policies and procedures. Most of the time, families find that their day care is open to working with them to set their child up for potty training success.

You'll want to be mindful of a few other things when it comes to potty training your child in day care. First, find out what kind of potty the day care uses and consider using the same one at home. Second, be sensitive to the needs of the day-care providers, as they are caring for multiple children at once and need to make practicality, hygiene, and cleanliness a priority. Third, be prepared for your child's day care to prefer pull-ups during nap times to avoid the extra cleanup from accidents. Fourth, always dress your child in practical clothing that's easy for your child to quickly remove during potty time in order to avoid accidents. And finally, provide the day care with at least two changes of pants, underwear, and socks.

You'll also want to pack a large waterproof bag in which to place soiled clothes.

If your child prefers a certain caregiver, ask if they're willing to lead the potty training responsibilities. This person would be in charge of watching for your child's signals, taking them to the potty each time, and handling accidents. If you've started the process at home, write down your child's unique signs and signals and potty patterns so that the caregiver is aware of them. Also, let your child know that when they need to go, they must let the caregiver know right away. You'll want to orient your child to the layout of the day care, including where the potty is located. Have them go on the potty prior to you leaving to help them feel comfortable.

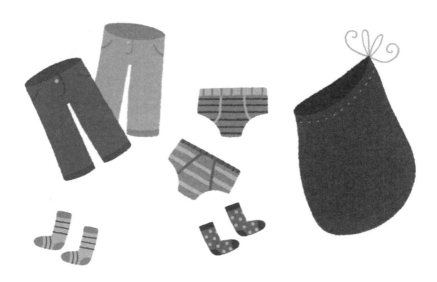

QUESTIONS TO ASK YOUR CHILD'S DAY-CARE PROVIDER:

▶ What is your system for taking children to the potty throughout the day? Do you prompt at certain times of the day or ask them if they need to go?

▶ How do you acknowledge children for using the potty? Do you give verbal praise or rewards or both?

▶ Do you put diapers on children who refuse to use the potty?

▶ How do you approach accidents?

▶ Do you record accidents throughout the day?

▶ What should I pack in my child's backpack for accidents?

▶ What is the procedure during nap times?

▶ Is it okay for my child to go commando the first couple of weeks of potty training?

Caregivers at Home

Many parents can't be involved in the potty training process 24/7 due to work schedules. Whether your child is with a day-care provider or stays with a caregiver at home, it's imperative to keep open communication with everyone involved. Ideally, you'll come up with a plan together before starting. Draw on the experience and expertise of your caregiver whenever possible. Collaborating and implementing their advice will make the training much easier.

Once you've started, check in with the caregiver on your child's daily successes and setbacks. Ask how the day went. Take some time once reunited with your child to convey how proud you are of them and encourage them to discuss their potty experiences without bombarding them with too many questions. You can say, "I would love to hear how going potty went for you today!" and allow them to share when they're ready.

Extended Family

Potty training works best when more than one adult is involved in the process. Not only is it helpful for your child to learn from different people, but it also relieves the pressure on the primary caregiver(s) if they have support.

When enlisting the support of extended family members, it's important to maintain open communication and collaborate as much as possible. Potty training must be a team effort when multiple caregivers are involved. If you've already started, share your strategies for what's been working well. Most will be happy to have a heads-up on what your experience has been so far—particularly regarding what works best for your child. If you're starting the journey together, come up with a united plan. From what clothing to wear, when (and if) to put on pull-ups, how to handle accidents, how often you're taking

Why Children Only Potty with Other Caregivers

Many parents report that their child uses the potty at day care but refuses to use it at home. One reason is because day cares often implement strict schedules that naturally incorporate potty breaks into the routine. They also tend to follow a potty routine that encourages children to be as independent as possible. For instance, your child may have to pull their pants down by themselves, wipe themselves, flush the toilet, wash and dry their hands, and return back to the group multiple times throughout the day. They may not have as consistent a routine at home, and every potty experience might be different, depending on the day, location, or caregiver. Too many variables can throw your child off track. Keep your child's routine as consistent as possible at home, and try to mimic the day care's routine.

Another reason for the discrepancy across environments is the caregiver's approach to reminders. Telling children that it's time to go potty, rather than asking if they need to go, is the best way to ensure compliance. Furthermore, day cares naturally incorporate positive peer pressure because they have the example of other children to follow. To remedy this, take your child to the bathroom with you as much as possible. Enlist support from other family members in this as well.

Children also trust you and know deep down there's nothing they can do to lose your love. Even if they feel comfortable in the care of others, your child may not place the same amount of trust in other caregivers. While your child likely feels safe with other providers, it's tempting for them to let loose and relax at home. There's no remedy for this situation other than to continue providing your child with unconditional love, even when they refuse to go potty or have accidents. Convey your confidence in your child and trust in the overall process.

planned trips to the potty, and whether to use rewards—make sure everyone is on the same page. And don't forget that all caregivers should emphasize the importance of fun, positivity, and patience.

Looking Back and Moving Forward

Let's recap the major points of this chapter:

▶ If you plan to enroll your child in day care, begin potty training at least 4 days before starting or shortly after your child has settled into their new environment. Potty training works best when other transitions and stress are eliminated.

▶ During your day-care interview, inquire about their potty training policies and procedures. Begin the dialogue early to ensure collaboration and consistency across all environments.

▶ If your child's day care will help while training, dress your child in easy-to-remove clothing and pack several changes of pants, underwear, and socks and a waterproof bag for soiled clothing. Also, let your child know who they can talk to when they need to go potty.

▶ Enlisting the support of extended family can be a huge help in the potty training journey. Not only is it great for your child to learn from different caregivers, but it also relieves some of the pressure on you.

▶ When involving extended family members, emphasize the importance of consistency across environments and caregivers. Share what's working for you if you've started potty training; if not, plan the process together.

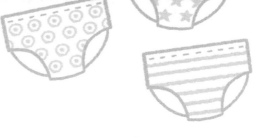

CHAPTER 8

Potty Training Away from Home

YOU AND YOUR CHILD will need to leave your home and your bathroom every now and then during potty training. Here's how to incorporate real life into your current surreal life.

Life Outside (and How to Include Potty Training)

At some point during the potty training process, you and your little one will need to leave your home. While it's tempting to stay inside, outings are a great way for your child to practice their new skills. In the early stages of potty training, keep your outings short and sweet in order to set your child up for success. (You'll gradually add in longer outings.) Here's what to keep in mind while potty training on the go.

Start Small

As noted earlier, your first few trips will be brief. For instance, take a walk around the block, make a quick visit to a family member's house, or run a short errand. Try to be gone for no more than 20 to 30 minutes at a time in the beginning, and have your child go potty right before leaving home. Don't go to appointments in the early days; putting your child on a time crunch and pressuring them to go potty quickly prior to leaving home will increase the likelihood of stress and accidents.

Prepare Your Child

Whether going to a new store or on an airplane, it's easy to forget how big the world feels to a young child. To minimize travel anxieties, help prepare them for the new environment. For instance, if you're visiting a new store, let your child know where the restrooms are and remind them to let you know if they need to use the potty. If you're going on a family vacation, show them pictures of where you're going and let them know all the things you plan to do while there. All of this will help your child feel more prepared for what's next and reduce the likelihood of accidents while on the go.

Stick with Your Potty Routine

Just because you're not home doesn't mean you ditch your potty routine. You'll want to maintain consistency, including the times at which you encourage your child to use the potty, the multiple steps involved in the routine (such as removing pants, wiping, flushing, and hand washing), and your reward system. There will be enough changes going on while traveling; try to stick with your potty routine as much as possible.

Dress for Success

Have your child wear easy-to-remove clothing that is stretchy and comfortable. Pants or shorts with elastic waists that are easy to push down and pull back up and dresses or skirts are ideal.

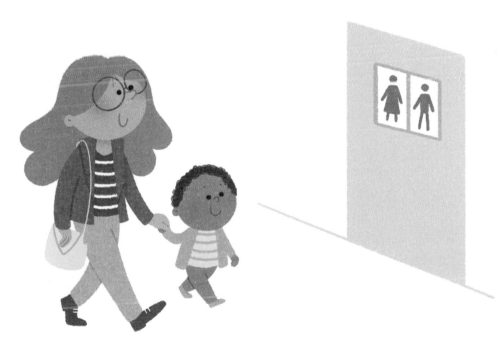

Bring Extra Clothes

Pack at least two changes of clothing (no matter how long your journey will be), including easy-to-remove pants or shorts (or skirts or dresses) and underwear. Keep in mind that your child may get urine on their socks and shoes if they have an accident, so bring extra socks and shoes as well. You'll also want to bring a waterproof bag for soiled clothing. Prep car seats and strollers with a waterproof cover in case of accidents.

WHAT TO BRING FOR OUTINGS:

▶ Two extra pairs of pants or shorts (or skirts or dresses) and underwear

▶ Extra pairs of socks and shoes

▶ Waterproof bag

▶ Waterproof covers for car seat and stroller

▶ Hand sanitizer

▶ Toilet paper

▶ Travel potty or toilet seat insert

▶ Towels for cleanup

Have the Travel Potty Ready to Go

It's not always possible to go to the restroom while on the go. Whether your child is not completely ready for public restrooms or you're visiting a place without a restroom (like parks and hiking trails), keep a travel potty in the car. A travel potty is more compact than a regular potty chair and is equipped for easy cleanup (it comes with plastic bags to discard after potty trips). Encourage your child to use it at home to get used to it. Say, "Let's pretend you're at the park and you need to go potty. What should you do? That's right! You'll let me know so that you can sit on this potty. Let's practice how you'll sit on it."

Handle Accidents with Patience

While in public, it's important to handle accidents the same way you would at home: with lots of patience. Help your child change into fresh clothes and enlist their help in cleaning up the mess. Use the same words you use at home, such as, "Oops. You had an accident in your pants. They are wet now. Remember, pee goes in the potty. Let's get you cleaned up."

Don't Avoid Public Toilets

Although it may seem daunting, try to conquer public toilets early on in the process. The faster your child gets used to them, the better off everyone will be. Accompany your child in the stall (of course), use the largest stall or family restroom when possible so that it's more comfortable, and bring a toilet insert. Make the process as fun as possible by singing, holding hands, and offering a small reward for a job well done. Prepare your child for the automatic flusher ahead of time by letting them know to expect a loud sound. Ideally, place something over the sensor (like a sticky note) so that you can control when it flushes. Use the restroom when you arrive at the store or when you leave the store (or both). This will help your child become more comfortable with public restrooms, and it will reduce the chance of accidents.

Visiting Friends and Family

Visiting friends and family often comes with added flexibility and comfort. For instance, you can bring your child's preferred potty chair and favorite potty books and toys to keep them occupied. Just be sure to give the host plenty of warning that you are potty training, and communicate how you prevent and handle accidents. They may want to prepare their home prior to your arrival. If you think it's necessary, you can also ask your friends and family to try to maintain a positive atmosphere for your child.

Travel

Traveling long distances in the early stages of potty training may seem daunting and stressful. It's best to have an established potty training routine (with lots of prior success) before going on family vacations. You want to be sure your child has mastered the basics before adding in other variables such as

Prompting Your On-the-Go Child

Your child is at risk for accidents while on the go because of distractions. They are often playing with other children or absorbed in activities, and you may be socializing. To help prevent accidents caused by distraction and forgetfulness, set a timer for 30 minutes to remind yourself to prompt your child to sit on the potty.

Children are often reluctant to go to the potty because they worry they'll miss out on something while on their potty break. Convey your understanding and reassure them patiently. Say, "I know you're having so much fun playing in the sandbox right now. It's time to go potty. The sandbox will be there when you get back." If they resist, offer two choices. Say, "It's time to go potty soon. Would you like to go in 2 minutes or 5 minutes?" Prompt them when the time comes, and always follow through with the trip to the potty, even if they resist. Encourage them to sit on the potty for a few minutes. Praise their compliance and potty success before taking them back to the fun. Once you return, reinforce the idea that the toys are still available to help minimize their resistance the next time. You can say something like, "Look! The toys were waiting for you to come back! Good job going potty. Now it's time to play."

new environments and busy schedules. Ideally, your child will have a month of potty training at home before going on vacation. However, this is not always possible, and vacationing while potty training can be done with added preparation and extra patience.

Vacations

When planning your family vacation with your newly trained child, consider staying in a place where you'll have access to laundry. It will come in handy during this phase! If this isn't possible, you can do laundry the old-fashioned way with detergent, a sink, and hangers to let the clothes air-dry. When picking your travel destination, try to be practical. Avoid traveling to places with long entrance lines, and opt for places with easy bathroom access. National parks and beach destinations are great go-tos during the early stages of potty training. Disney parks are also popular due to their baby care centers that have kid-sized toilets and lower sinks for little ones to wash their hands.

Air Travel

If you're considering long-distance travel, you'll need to get your child accustomed to using public restrooms. After all, they will likely have to go at the airport, on the airplane, and in hotels and restaurants. Unless you want to (and are able to) carry a travel potty with you everywhere, your child will need to be comfortable with public restrooms prior to traveling.

When booking your flight, try to sit on the aisle to make it easy for your child to go to the restroom. Once you arrive at the airport, have your child try to go potty even if they insist they don't need to go. Long airport security lines and distant gates will increase the likelihood of your child needing to go at inopportune times.

It's okay to put your child in a pull-up during long flights. There will be several times during the trip when going to the potty will be impossible, such as during takeoff, turbulence, and traveling to the gate. Just be sure to explain to your child why you're using the pull-up, and do not use the word *diaper*. If you're afraid of regression, place underwear underneath the pull-up so that they can feel the wetness. Tell your child to keep their underwear dry and to let you know when they need to go potty. Praise them if they are able to do so. Try to take your child to the restroom as soon as the seat belt light goes off, and give your child a heads-up about the loud toilet flush. Have them stand outside the restroom while you flush since airplane toilet flushes tend to be exceptionally loud. Visit the restroom regularly during the flight (just as you would at home or other places), and remove their pull-up as soon as you get off the plane (or as soon as you reach your destination if you anticipate long travel times).

Car Trips

When planning your road trip, map out rest areas and other places you can stop for a potty break. While it's not always

What to Bring While On the Go

- At least two changes of pants or shorts (or skirts or dresses) and underwear

- Extra socks and shoes

- A sticky note for public toilets with automatic flushers

- Waterproof bag for soiled clothes

- Travel potty

- Toilet insert for public restrooms

- Wipes

- Bag for dirty wipes

- Hand sanitizer

- Extra pull-ups (for naptime and bedtime)

- Must-have potty toys

- Waterproof covers for car seat and stroller

- Laundry detergent (for vacations)

- Mattress covers (if night training)

- Small rewards (if applicable)

- Small towel to wipe up messes

possible, try to limit drinks an hour before leaving home if you're planning a long car ride to help prevent accidents in the car. Also, plan frequent, regularly scheduled stops (every hour or so) to give your child plenty of opportunities to go. Like airplane rides, it's okay to put your child in a pull-up for long car rides. (Follow the guidelines above for using a pull-up on the airplane.) Once you arrive at your destination, remove the pull-up.

It can be hectic to manage potty training while on the go, but it can be done. A little preparation and an extra dose of patience will go a long way. Also, be prepared for regression after you return from family vacations, especially if the potty training schedule was lax while you were away. If this is the case, get back to your potty routine and reward system as soon as you get home. You may also need to return to the basics like potty books and play. You should see the situation return to normal in a few days.

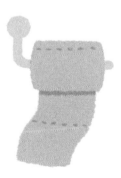

Looking Back and Moving Forward

Let's recap the major points of this chapter:

▶ Traveling early on in the potty training process can seem daunting, but it can be done.

▶ Ideally, your child will have mastered potty training at home before going on long family vacations.

▶ Whether you are traveling around town or far away, be prepared for accidents by bringing extra changes of clothes, a travel potty, a toilet insert, wipes, treats (if applicable), and other potty necessities.

▶ Prepare your child for what to expect when traveling.

▶ Stick with your potty routine as much as possible while on the go. That means maintaining consistency in terms of common times your child goes to the potty and continuing to reward them with small treats (if applicable).

▶ Try to give your child lots of practice using public restrooms before going on vacation.

▶ Prepare your family and friends prior to your arrival by letting them know you're potty training. Tell them how you prevent and manage accidents, and encourage a positive atmosphere as much as possible.

▶ Set a timer for every 30 minutes to remind yourself to prompt your child to go potty, and choose your prompting language carefully.

▶ Don't be afraid to put your child in pull-ups during airplane rides and long road trips. If you fear regression, place underwear underneath their pull-up so they can feel the wetness. Just be sure to remove the pull-up and go back to the potty routine as soon as possible.

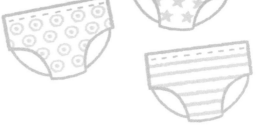

CHAPTER 9

Troubleshooting

EVEN THE BEST-LAID PLANS CAN FAIL, through no fault of your own or your child. In fact, more than 80 percent of children will experience setbacks while potty training—whether you're a first-time parent or not. This means that what we refer to as "setbacks" are just par for the course when it comes to potty training. Here are some common setbacks and strategies to help.

Diarrhea and Constipation

Issues with bowel movements, like constipation and diarrhea, can slow down the progress of potty training. It's important to remedy these situations before continuing.

Diarrhea

If your child is sick and has diarrhea, the best thing you can do is to rediaper and start again once they're feeling better. Your child will have an extremely hard time trying to learn when they're sick. It's all beyond their control.

If your child has diarrhea, encourage them to drink lots of fluids, particularly water, to prevent dehydration. Feed them starchy foods, like cereals, grains, rice, pasta, crackers, and mashed potatoes, because they're easy to digest. Soft-boiled eggs and yogurt are also easily digested and will add protein to your child's diet. Saltine crackers and pretzels can meet your child's need for sodium. If your child has mild diarrhea, avoid fruit juices and carbonated drinks and limit beans and other foods that cause loose stools. Resume potty training once your child's diarrhea has completely subsided and they are back in good health.

Constipation

Constipation is a very subtle, yet powerful, obstacle to potty training that has less to do with how often your child poops and more to do with how hard the poop is when it comes out. The ideal poop has the consistency of toothpaste or hummus, and anything else is technically constipation to some degree. You'll know your child is experiencing constipation if they begin to poop less often (fewer than three times per week) and their bowel movements are hard, pebbly, and difficult to push out. Constipation can lead to potty avoidance because bowel movements become painful to pass.

Constipation means poop is trapped in the colon, which stretches the bowel. The job of the colon is to absorb the water from the poop to prevent diarrhea. The longer poop is in the colon, the more water is absorbed, making the poop harder. As poop accumulates in the colon, it begins to block the nerve signals between the abdomen and the brain. When these signals are blocked, it becomes difficult for your child to feel if they have to urinate or defecate, making accidents more common.

In severe cases, children can have impacted poop, which causes a plug in the bowel. When this is the case, you will notice loose, watery smears in their pull-ups or underwear. This is a sign of serious constipation, and your child should be assessed and treated by their pediatrician. In less severe cases, you can treat constipation with home remedies such as exercising, taking warm baths, and adjusting their diet.

You'll want to load up your child on dried or fresh fruits such mango, pineapple, papaya, berries, pears, peaches, plums, and apples. Two to four ounces of pear or prune juice a day can also help reduce constipation. Consider other fiber-rich foods like vegetables (such as broccoli or peas), beans, and whole-grain cereals and breads. Make sure your child drinks plenty of fluids and exercises regularly. You'll also want to cut back on bananas and high-iron foods like rice and Cheerios because these foods can be constipating. Processed grains, like white bread, white rice, and white pastas and dairy products are also known to cause constipation. Hold off on potty training until your child's stool is consistently a mushy texture (like toothpaste).

COMMON SIGNS OF CONSTIPATION:

▶ Feces the consistency of pebbles (hard, dry, and lumpy)

▶ Bowel movements appear painful and difficult to pass (your child cries and screams during bowel movements)

▶ Your child avoids or resists potty trips by clenching their buttocks, turning red, running away, crossing their legs, or crying and screaming

▶ Less than three bowel movements per week

▶ Complaints of stomachaches

▶ Abdominal swelling

▶ Rectal bleeding

▶ Frequent urination and/or accidents

▶ Liquid or smears of stool in underwear

Temper Tantrums

Early childhood and tantrums seem to go hand in hand. Meltdowns are extremely common at this age due to your child's limited vocabulary to express their emotions and their strong desire to assert their independence. And potty training is a huge transition that comes with some degree of stress, which can cause tantrums.

Try not to view tantrums as defiance; think of them as a way for your child to communicate with you. When your child starts throwing a tantrum, try to identify their underlying feelings and potential unmet needs. For instance, are they hungry, tired, lonely, or overstimulated, or are they trying to tell you that they're stressed about this whole potty thing? Maybe they're letting you know that your approach to potty training feels like a threat to their independence. Try to decode the thoughts and feelings behind your child's behavior, but be aware that you won't always be sure of the underlying cause of the tantrum—and that's okay. The most important thing is to understand that your child is signaling an unmet need or desire, so view tantrums as your child's way of communicating with you.

Stay Connected

The quickest way to return to baseline during tantrums is to connect with your child emotionally. Get down on their level, make eye contact, offer physical touch (but pull back if they tell you they don't want to be touched), acknowledge their feelings, and avoid asking questions or making comments. It's okay if you don't fully understand what they are trying to tell you; simply identify and validate their emotions. Less is more during tantrums, so now is not the time to have a rational conversation with your child. They simply cannot register logical ideas when they're in the middle of a tantrum. Stay close and wait it out. While you wait, take note of triggers and possible underlying needs. This is a great time to have an honest look at your potty training approach and any recent stressors in your child's life. For instance, have you been using punishments, such as threats and yelling? Are they experiencing any other transitions at this time? Has your overall training approach been consistent? Consider whether a simple adjustment to your teaching technique might make your child feel more at ease.

Take a Short Break

Tantrums are inopportune times to teach your child new skills. Think about taking a brief break if your child is

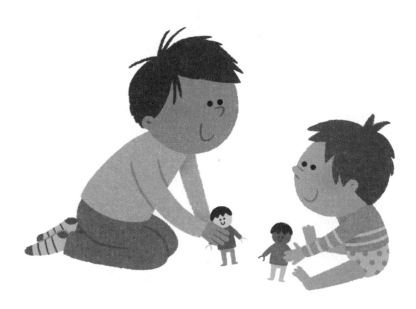

having tantrums throughout the day, nearly every day. You can resume later in the day or the next day. Use the time off to focus on connecting with your child. Play their favorite games, and get them involved in other activities to help reduce stress. Reintroduce fun by reading potty training books and watching related videos. Also, use this time to play out potty training scenes and process any potty-related anxiety.

Empathize

What if you determine your child is physically and psychologically ready and your approach has been consistent, predictable, and positive? If your child has potty training tantrums, try to relax and stay as neutral and casual about potty training as you possibly can. Listen to your child's comments and empathize with their concerns. Try to understand potty training from their perspective. Say that you understand how difficult going to the potty can be and that you're supporting them every step of the way. Discuss your child's worries and self-doubts openly to help them process their feelings.

If they tantrum while on the potty, say, "I see that you're upset right now. I really appreciate you sitting on the potty and trying to go." If your child sits on the potty and does not go, simply thank them for trying and let them know you'll try again later.

Take a Longer Break

Temper tantrums may be a sign power struggles have begun. Here's the thing about potty training that you must never lose sight of: fights with your child about their body are battles you will never win. Your child has to *want* to go potty in order for potty training to be successful. When children feel pressured and forced to go potty, they begin to resist in order to assert their control over their bodies.

If your child refuses to go on the potty and has frequent tantrums over it, it may be time to take a longer break to reevaluate your child's developmental readiness and your overall approach. Review what works and doesn't work about your training approach, make plans for adjustment, and try again at a later time. Remember, your child may be physically able to potty train, but may not be psychologically ready. Your child *must* be an excited, motivated, and curious participant.

In general, try to think of breaks like this as a last resort, and don't take more than one day off if possible. Here's the thing with breaks: they can set you back because you and your child will have to reestablish a potty routine. Frequent starts and stops can also make your child feel confused, which can lead to even more resistance. Besides, you don't want to send the message that tantrums mean getting what they want (breaks from potty training).

If your child continues to be resistant or disinterested in the potty for the first *several weeks* of the process, your child may not be developmentally ready for potty training. Take a break and start again at a later time.

IF YOUR CHILD DISPLAYS SOME OF THESE SIGNS FOR SEVERAL WEEKS, IT MAY BE TIME TO HOLD OFF ON POTTY TRAINING:

▶ Your child has several accidents in a row for multiple days and never makes an attempt to get to the potty

▶ Your child starts hiding during their accidents

▶ Your child repeatedly refuses to sit on the toilet

Get Help

Don't be afraid to reach out for professional advice if you notice frequent power struggles. Your child's behavior may be a symptom of an underlying problem, such as relational issues between you and your child, a mental health issue such as ADHD, anxiety, or depression, or a developmental disorder. A psychologist or family therapist will be able to offer a fresh perspective and new insights into the issue(s).

Regressive Behaviors

So potty training was a success for a while, but now your child is displaying regressive behaviors, such as demanding you put their diapers back on or insisting they're still a baby. This is common behavior in young children, especially those with younger siblings, who still want to be a baby in your eyes. To ease their fear, tell them that they will always be your baby no matter how old they are.

Also, be mindful of your approach to praising, as excessive compliments can inadvertently cause your child to feel pressured to perform well and never make mistakes. You don't want your child to feel like they've let you down when they have an accident. Instead, offer genuine and simple praises such as "I'm so proud of you!" and a hug or high five. The most powerful help we can offer our children when potty training is our faith that it will happen. Relax and offer support, even when your child displays regressive behaviors. (And it may help to know that most regressions subside within 2 weeks.)

Here are more strategies to keep in mind if your child is demonstrating regressive behaviors:

▶ **MAINTAIN A CONSISTENT ROUTINE.**
Always incorporate a regular potty schedule into your daily routine. Prompt your child to go to the potty before and after transitions, and have them

sit on the potty shortly after waking up and after every meal. Children thrive on routine and feel safer and content when they know what to expect from their environment.

▶ **GO BACK TO THE BASICS.** If the accidents are constant, return to the basics of when you first started, including reading potty books, going naked, and receiving rewards for a job well done.

▶ **STAY POSITIVE.** Don't show disappointment and disapproval when your child has accidents. Your frustration can increase your child's anxiety, which in turn can lead to more potty problems. Try to be positive, nonjudgmental, and matter-of-fact. You can say something like, "Oops, you had an accident. Let's go sit on the potty." After they are done, involve them in the cleanup process. Praise your child for helping you clean up and move on.

▶ **GIVE EXTRA TLC.** Regressions are stressful not only for you, but also for your child. They want to know there's nothing they can do to lose your love, so offer your child lots of attention and as much one-on-one time during regressions as possible, especially if there is a new baby at home or other family changes. Sit with your child while they use the potty (if they feel comfortable) or eat. Make time to get down on their level and play with them, even if it's just for 10 minutes. Regular one-on-one attention throughout the day can help prevent accidents.

Backsliding into Accidents

It's not uncommon for children to appear to have mastered potty training only to start having accidents. It's important to determine whether your child has truly regressed or if they're having accidents that are par for the course in the early stages of potty training. Either way, occasional setbacks in the early days, months, and even years of potty training are normal.

When your child begins to backslide into accidents, try not to panic. You'll need to determine the underlying causes of their frequent accidents so that you can begin to prevent them. Here are some common reasons your child might be backsliding into accidents and some simple solutions.

Your Child Isn't Ready

When your child starts having more accidents than potty successes, it's time to take an honest look at whether they are developmentally ready. Your child must be both physically and emotionally ready for potty training to be a success. They must have a strong urge toward independence and self-mastery. Don't be afraid to set the potty aside for a while if you get the sense they are overwhelmed by potty training. (Keep in mind, though, that it's usually best to continue moving forward, however gradually, especially if you've determined your child is developmentally ready for potty training.)

Constipation and Other Medical Issues

As mentioned earlier, constipation is a common cause of accidents because the blocked stool interferes with nerve signals from the abdomen to the brain, preventing your child from knowing when they have to go to the potty. Constipation is also extremely painful, so children will naturally avoid going to the potty in order to prevent discomfort. Your child may also steer clear of the potty if they are experiencing medical issues like a urinary tract or intestinal infection. Be sure to rule out any medical issues with your child's pediatrician before proceeding with potty training.

Your Child Is Distracted

Sometimes accidents happen because your child is distracted or doesn't want to give up a beloved toy or activity. When this is the case, they are more likely to have an accident because they wait until the last minute or don't make it to the bathroom. It's very common for young children to prefer playing to going to the potty. When this is the case, prompt your child to go potty before they begin playing, and give them extra reminders if needed. Follow your child's lead and go with their preferred method.

Stress and Transitions

Stress is another common cause of accidents. When your child is stressed from changes in their environment, it's hard for them to concentrate on learning new skills, such as potty training. If your child feels embarrassed and ashamed for having an accident at school or in public, this, too, can cause them to be more susceptible to accidents. In older children, it's not uncommon to see more frequent accidents when they feel they don't have much control over their environment. You'll want to understand the root of their stress in order to help them overcome it.

Starting Late

The age at which your child begins potty training is highly variable. Truth be told, the age to start potty training is all over the map. Whether you delayed potty training due to your child's development, medical issues, family stressors, or because you simply were not ready, it's going to be okay. Your child will learn to be potty trained even if they start a little later than other children.

What If I Want to Give Up?

It's no secret that potty training can be tough—especially when you've never done it before! Whether it's the frequent accidents, constant power struggles, or relentless constipation, potty training is hard work. Deciding whether to stop potty training is a personal decision that only you can make. It's important to weigh the pros and cons of taking a break, discuss the decision with other involved caregivers, and then trust your intuition. You know what's best for you and your child, and only you can make that decision. You are always free to change your mind.

If you tough it out and continue, you could very well see the light at the end of the tunnel soon and achieve wonderful potty success Imagine the level of con-

fidence and pride you will feel knowing you toughed it out and saw it through! On the other hand, not taking a break can take a toll on your parent–child relationship if you are constantly having power struggles and negative experiences with potty training in general. Your break from potty training could be what you both need.

If you feel the urge to quit is due to your own exhaustion and frustration, enlist the support of a friend or family member to help you. Try to get enough support so that you can take a brief break before you stop the process altogether. On the other hand, if your desire to stop is mainly from your child's resistance, you may want to take a breather and reevaluate their developmental readiness.

Potty training later comes with its own advantages and disadvantages. Training late is associated with higher risk of constipation and withholding poop. You may also find that your older child is more resistant to letting go of their diapers because they are more stuck in their ways. On the other hand, starting late means that your child is much more likely to be aware of their body's signals that it's time to go. They are more physically capable of dressing and undressing independently and wiping reasonably well. At an older age, they are also more likely to feel peer pressure when they find out their friends are already trained; this may prompt them to train more quickly themselves.

Whether or not you've decided to train later, the strategies for older children will be the same as those for younger children. In addition, you'll want to avoid shaming your child into becoming a big kid and comparing them to their siblings and friends. Avoid pushing too hard or too fast. Most of all, relax into it. You may feel you need to get your child fully potty trained quickly, but try your best not to put pressure on yourself and your child. Your job is to set the conditions that make it easier for your child to go and leave the rest up to them. Ultimately, your child will be toilet trained.

Looking Back and Moving Forward

Let's recap the major points of this chapter:

▶ Medical issues such as diarrhea and constipation are common roadblocks in the potty training process. While severe diarrhea may require a break, you can continue training through mild constipation and diarrhea with the help of home remedies.

▶ Consult with your child's pediatrician if you're concerned medical issues are impeding potty training.

▶ While tantrums and pushback are common, there are things you can do to reconnect with your child and minimize resistance. If tantrums have become constant, reevaluate your child's readiness for potty training, possible stressors, and your overall approach to the process.

▶ Regressive behaviors are common among younger children, especially if they have a new sibling. Reevaluate your approach to praise, especially if you suspect it's causing too much pressure to perform.

▶ Try not to panic when your child begins backsliding into accidents. Instead, establish and maintain a consistent routine, go back to the basics, stay positive, and give your child lots of extra attention. Most regressions subside within 2 weeks.

▶ Late training comes with its own set of advantages and disadvantages. Resist the urge to pressure your child into accomplishing this quickly or comparing them to other children.

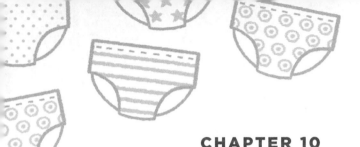

CHAPTER 10

Celebrate!

WOW, SO YOU AND YOUR CHILD ARE DONE?
You've read this book, followed the strategies, made the adjustments necessary to tailor the journey to your child, and now you're finished! You officially have a diaper-free child on your hands. Your child has figured out that clean, dry underwear is far better than soggy diapers and puddles on the floor. Fantastic work! I know there were many highs and lows, successes and failures, accidents and potty celebrations along the way. I'm sure you're both excited and a little bit tired from the journey. There may have been times you wanted to give up, asking yourself, *Is my child ready for this? Heck, am I ready for this?* But you made it! What a huge accomplishment both for you and your child. Potty training is one of your child's biggest developmental milestones, and you were their biggest supporter along the way. This calls for one last potty dance party to celebrate!

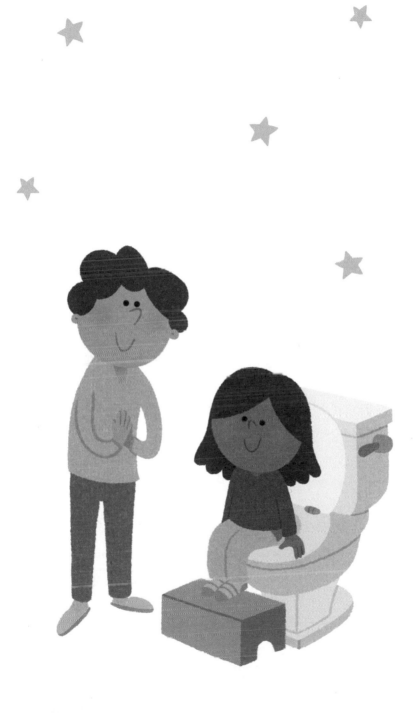

Resources

General Children's Potty Books

- *Daniel's Potty Time* by Daniel Tiger's Neighborhood

- *Potty* by Leslie Patricelli

- *P Is for Potty!* (Sesame Street) by Naomi Kleinberg

- *The Potty Book: For Girls* (Hannah & Henry Series) by Alyssa Satin Capucilli

- *The Potty Book: For Boys* (Hannah & Henry Series) by Alyssa Satin Capucilli

- *Big Girl Panties* by Fran Manushkin

- *Princess Potty* by Samantha Berger and Amy Cartwright

- *Potty Superhero: Get Ready for Big Boy Pants!* by Parragon Books

- *A Potty for Me!* by Karen Katz

- *Once Upon a Potty: Girl* by Alona Frankel

- *Once Upon a Potty: Boy* by Alona Frankel

Children's Books on Pooping

- *It Hurts When I Poop! A Story for Children Who Are Scared to Use the Potty* by Howard J. Bennett, MD

- *Where's the Poop?* by Julie Markes

- *The Potty Train* by David Hochman

- *Everyone Poops* by Taro Gomi

- *"Bloop, Bloop!" Goes the Poop* by Temara Moore

Educational DVDs about Potty Training

- *Sesame Street: Elmo's Potty Time*

- *Bear in the Big Blue House: Potty Time with Bear*

- PBS KIDS, *It's Potty Time*

- *Potty Power: For Boys & Girls*

- *Once Upon a Potty: For Her* [or *For Him*]

Children's Anatomy Books

- *Little Explorers: My Amazing Body* by Ruth Martin

- *Inside Your Outside: All About the Human Body* by Tish Rabe

- *Who Has What? All About Girls' Bodies and Boys' Bodies* by Robie H. Harris

References

American Academy of Pediatrics. "Practice Guide: Toilet Training." Accessed on December 17, 2019, www.aap.org/en-us/advocacy-and-policy/aap-health-initiatives/practicing-safety/Documents/ToiletTraining.pdf.

American Academy of Pediatrics. "Toilet Training." Accessed on December 17, 2019, www.aap.org/en-us/advocacy-and-policy/aap-health-initiatives/practicing-safety/Pages/Toilet-Training.aspx.

American Academy of Pediatrics. "Toilet Training Guidelines: Day Care Providers—The Role of the Day Care Provider in Toilet Training." *Pediatrics* 103, Supplement 3 (1999): 1367-1368. Accessed December 19, 2019, https://pediatrics.aappublications.org/content/103/Supplement_3/1367/tab-article-info.

American Academy of Pediatrics. "Toilet Training Guidelines: The Role of Parents in Toilet Training." *Pediatrics* 103, no. 6 (1999): 1362–1363.

Brown, F., and N. Peace. "Teaching a Child with Challenging Behavior to Use the Toilet: A Clinical Case Study." *British Journal of Learning Disabilities* 39 (2011): 321–326. https://onlinelibrary.wiley .com/doi/abs/10.1111/j.1468-3156.2011.00676.x.

Choby, B., and S. George. "Toilet Training." *American Family Physician* 78, no. 9 (2008): 1059–1064.

Connell-Carrick, K. "Trends in Popular Parenting Books and the Need for Parental Critical Thinking." *Child Welfare* 85, no. 5 (2006): 819–836.

Doan, D., and K. Toussaint. "A Parent-Oriented Approach to Rapid Toilet Training." *International Electronic Journal of Elementary Education* 9, no. 2 (2016): 473–486.

Greer, B., P. Neidert, and C. Dozier. "A Component Analysis of Toilet-Training Procedures Recommended for Young Children." *Journal of Applied Behavior Analysis* 49, no. 1 (2015): 69–84. https://doi.org/10.1002/jaba.275.

Harlan, G. "When is the best time to toilet train?" *Journal Watch Psychiatry* (2003). https://doi:10.1056/jp200307090000010.

HealthyChildren.org. "Praise and Reward Your Child's Success." (2009). Accessed on December 17, 2019, www .healthychildren.org/English/ages-stages/toddler/toilet-training/ Pages/Praise-and-Reward-Your-Childs-Success.aspx.

InformedHealth.org. "Bedwetting: Overview." (2006). Accessed February 17, 2020, www.ncbi.nlm.nih.gov/books/NBK279494/.

Kiddoo, D. "Toilet Training Children: When to Start and How to Train." *Canadian Medical Association* 184, no. 5 (2012): 511–512.

Kimball, V. "The Perils and Pitfalls of Potty Training." *Pediatrics Annals* 45, no. 6 (2016):199–201. https://doi:10.3928/00904481-20160512-01.

Kinservik, M., and M. Friedhoff. "Control Issues in Toilet Training." *Pediatric Nursing* 26, no. 3 (2000): 267–272.

Mayo Clinic. "Bed-Wetting." Accessed February 17, 2020, www.mayoclinic.org/diseases-conditions/bed-wetting/symptoms-causes/syc-20366685.

Meyerhoff, M. "Perspectives on Parenting: Toilet Training Tips." *Pediatrics for Parents* 31, nos. 5–6 (2010): 8–9.

Mruzek, D., B. Handen, C. Aponte, T. Smith, and R. Foxx. "Parent Training for Toileting in Autism Spectrum Disorder." *American Psychological Association* (2019): 203–230. http://dx.doi.org/10.1037/0000111-009.

Parker-Pope, T. "Dr. T. Berry Brazelton on Naps and Toilet Time." *New York Times.* September 17, 2008. Accessed on December 19, 2019, https://well.blogs.nytimes.com/2008/09/17/dr-t-berry-brazelton-on-naps-and-toilet-time/.

Ritblatt, S., A. Obegi, B. Hammons, T. Ganger, and B. Ganger. "Parents' and Child Care Professionals' Toilet Training Attitudes and Practices: A Comparative Analysis." *Journal of Research in Childhood Education* 17, no. 2 (2003): 133–146.

Russell, K. "Among Healthy Children, What Toilet-Training Strategy Is Most Effective and Prevents Fewer Adverse Events (Stool withholding and Dysfunctional Voiding)?" *Pediatric Child Health* 13, no. 3 (2008): 201–202.

Schmitt, B. "Toilet Training Your Child: The Basics." *Contemporary Pediatrics* 21, no. 3 (2004): 120–122.

Simon, J., and R. Thompson. "The Effects of Undergarment Type on Urinary Continence of Toddlers." *Journal of Applied Behavior Analysis* 39, no. 3 (2006): 363–368. https://doi:10.1901/jaba.2006.124-05.

Index

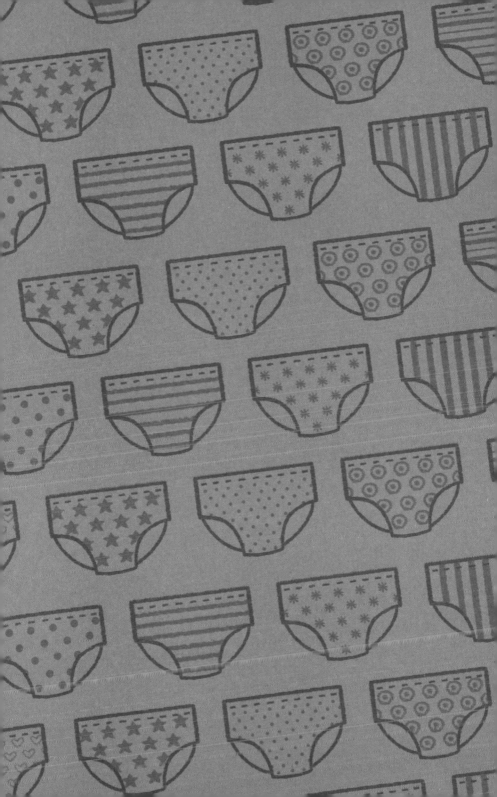

Acknowledgments

As a clinical psychologist and mother of two children, I understand how challenging parenting can be. I also know how important encouragement and practical advice are when encountering huge milestones, such as potty training. I wrote this book for busy, first-time parents who are in search of straightforward and practical information on potty training. My hope is to teach you the potty training basics while offering support and encouragement every step of the way.

Without a doubt, I would not have written this book without the support and accountability provided by Penguin Random House, especially Susan Randol and Meg Ilasco. Thank you for such an amazing opportunity.

This book is dedicated to my loving husband, Jessie, and our two beautiful daughters, Jaliyah and Jayla. I am so incredibly thankful for you all. Thank you for making me feel like the luckiest woman alive each and every day.

About the Author

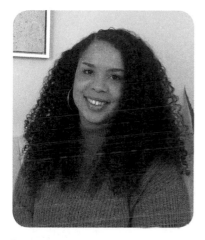

DR. JAZMINE McCOY is a clinical psychologist and the mother of two daughters: Jaliyah and Jayla. She specializes in parenting, child development, and maternal mental health. Through her work with children and families in her private practice and her online community, Dr. Jazmine is committed to helping overwhelmed and exhausted parents understand and connect with their children, despite their difficult and confusing behaviors. She offers courses, books, and educational videos on her website to help guide parents through the process of raising happy, resilient, and respectful children. She resides with her husband, two children, and small dog, Valentino, in the Sacramento, California area.

Join her online community for education and support on parenting, child development, and maternal mental health.

WEBSITE: www.themompsychologist.com
AMAZON: http://amazon.com/author/jazminemccoy
FACEBOOK: www.facebook.com/themompsychologist
INSTAGRAM: www.instagram.com/themompsychologist
YOUTUBE: www.youtube.com/c/themompsychologist

Hi there!

We hope this book was helpful in your potty training journey. Dr. Jazmine is offering bonus content to help with your little one, including checklists, practical guides, and more. Sign up for Dr. Jazmine's newsletter by December 31, 2021 to access these extras for free by going to **www.themompsychologist.com/pottytraining**.

Please consider writing a review on your favorite retailer's website to let others know what you thought of the book! Also, don't hesitate to reach out to **customerservice@penguinrandomhouse.com** if you have any questions or concerns about your book. We're here and happy to help.

Sincerely,

Zeitgeist Publishing